HOW THE MIND WORKS

HOW THE MIND WORKS

Concepts and Cases in Psychoanalysis and Psychotherapy

Kevin Volkan and Vamık Volkan

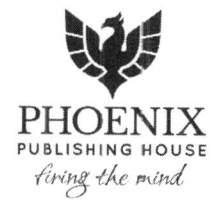

PHOENIX
PUBLISHING HOUSE
firing the mind

First published in 2023 by
Phoenix Publishing House Ltd
62 Bucknell Road
Bicester
Oxfordshire OX26 2DS

British Library Cataloguing in Publication Data

A C.I.P. for this book is available from the British Library

ISBN-13: 978-1-80013-199-6

Typeset by vPrompt eServices Pvt Ltd, India

Printed in the United Kingdom

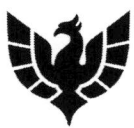

www.firingthemind.com

Contents

About the authors

Kevin Volkan, EdD, PhD, MPH is a founding faculty member and professor of psychology at California State University Channel Islands, where he researches and teaches courses on psychopathology and atypical behaviors, personality theory, as well as Nazi Germany and Eastern philosophy. Dr. Volkan also currently serves on the Graduate Medical Education faculty for the Community Memorial Hospital System in Ventura, CA, where he teaches and conducts research with medical residents, and as Adjunct Professor of Clinical Psychology in California Lutheran University's clinical psychology doctorate program.

He holds doctorates in clinical and quantitative psychology and is a graduate of the Harvard School of Public Health and a former Harvard Medical School faculty member and administrator. Dr. Volkan is an expert on extreme psychopathologies and has testified before the United States Senate on pathological and dangerous fetishes. He serves as a forensic psychology consultant to both state and federal law enforcement agencies. Dr. Volkan has made numerous appearances on television, radio, and podcasts as a psychological expert.

Although Dr. Volkan's clinical training and experience is in psycho-analytic psychotherapy, he has used other modalities in clinical practice. He has practiced clinical psychology as a staff psychologist in a state hospital and in private practice. Dr. Volkan's clients included a diverse population of people representing a wide variety of socioeconomic strata and psychological distress. He has worked with people suffering from drug addiction, neuroses, and personality disorders as well as individuals suffering from autism, organic brain injury, and schizophrenia. Dr. Volkan was awarded the Sustained Superior Accomplishment Award from the State of California for his clinical work. His current practice is centered upon psychodynamic embodied dreamwork.

Vamık Volkan, MD, DFLAPA, was born to Turkish parents in Cyprus. Before coming to the United States in 1957 he received his medical education at the School of Medicine, University of Ankara, Turkey.

He is an emeritus professor of psychiatry at the University of Virginia, Charlottesville, Virginia and an emeritus training and supervising analyst at the Washington Baltimore Psychoanalytic Center.

For eighteen of his thirty-nine years at the University of Virginia, Dr. Volkan was the medical director of the University's Blue Ridge Hospital. In 1987, he established the Center for the Study of Mind and Human Interaction (CSMHI). CSMHI applied a growing theoretical and field-proven base of knowledge to issues such as ethnic tension, racism, large-group identity, terrorism, societal trauma, immigration, mourning, transgenerational transmissions, leader–follower relationships, and other aspects of national and international conflict.

A year after his 2002 retirement, Dr. Volkan became the Senior Erik Erikson Scholar at the Erikson Institute of the Austen Riggs Center in Stockbridge, Massachusetts for ten years.

Dr. Volkan is a former president of the Turkish-American Neuropsychiatric Society, the International Society of Political Psychology, the Virginia Psychoanalytic Society, and the American College of Psychoanalysts.

He was an inaugural Yitzhak Rabin Fellow at the Rabin Center, Tel Aviv, Israel; a visiting professor of law at Harvard University, Boston, Massachusetts; a visiting professor of political science at the University of Vienna, Vienna, Austria and at Bahçeşehir University, Istanbul, Turkey. He worked as a visiting professor of psychiatry at three universities in

Turkey. In 2006, he was Fulbright/Sigmund Freud-Privatstiftung Visiting Scholar of Psychoanalysis in Vienna, Austria. In 2015, he became a visiting professor at El Bosque University, Bogota, Colombia.

Dr. Volkan holds honorary doctorate degrees from Kuopio University (now called the University of Eastern Finland), Finland; from Ankara University, Turkey; and the Eastern European Psychoanalytic Institute, Russia. He was a member of the Working Group on Terror and Terrorism, International Psychoanalytical Association. He was a temporary consultant to the World Health Organization (WHO) in Albania and Macedonia.

He received the Nevitt Sanford Award, Elise M. Hayman Award, L. Bryce Boyer Award, Margaret Mahler Literature Prize, Hans H. Strupp Award, and American College of Psychoanalysts' Distinguished Officer Award for 2014 and Gravida 2021 Best Book Award. He also received the Sigmund Freud Award given by the city of Vienna, Austria in collaboration with the World Council of Psychotherapy and the Mary S. Sigourney Award for 2015. The Sigourney Award was given to him for his role as a "seminal contributor to the application of psychoanalytic thinking to conflicts between countries and cultures," and because "his clinical thinking about the use of object relations theory in primitive mental states has advanced our understanding of severe personality disorders." He also was honored on several occasions by being nominated for the Nobel Peace Prize, with letters of support from twenty-seven countries.

Dr. Volkan is the author, coauthor, editor, or coeditor of sixty-two psychoanalytic and psychopolitical books, some of which have been translated into Turkish, Finnish, German, Serbian, Spanish, Chinese, Portuguese, Russian, Japanese, and Greek. He has written hundreds of published papers and book chapters. He has served on the editorial boards of sixteen national or international professional journals, including the *Journal of the American Psychoanalytic Association*, and was the guest editor of the Diamond Jubilee Special Issue of the *American Journal of Psychoanalysis*, 2015.

Dr. Volkan continues to lecture nationally and internationally.

About this book

In the literature related to helping people to have a more comfortable mental state, we see references to many types of psychotherapies, such as supportive therapy, cognitive behavior therapy, dialectical behavior therapy, existential therapy, aversion therapy, Gestalt therapy, hypnotherapy, art therapy, systematic desensitization, psychodrama, family therapy, marriage therapy, group therapy, and even nude therapy. This book examines and describes psychoanalytic concepts, psychoanalytic psychotherapy (sometimes called psychodynamic psychotherapy, dynamic psychotherapy, or insight therapy), and psychoanalytic group therapy.

Over a decade ago, based on decades-long clinical experiences starting in the early 1960s, Vamık Volkan published a textbook on psychoanalytic treatment that includes stories of psychoanalytic processes from the first to the last day of treatments of various types of analysands (V. D. Volkan, 2010). He has also written other books of psychoanalytic cases spanning the first to the last days of psychoanalysis and reporting what comes to the psychoanalyst's mind—and when cases were supervised, also the supervisor's mind—as the analytic process continued (V. D. Volkan, 2005, 2010, 2013, 2019a, 2019b, 2021a, 2021b; V. D. Volkan & Fowler, 2009). Writing total case histories allows the reader to question the validity of the link between clinical observations, the psychodynamic understanding of them, and technical considerations based on such observations. The best way to describe major changes in a person's internal world, we believe, is to recount total psychoanalytic processes.

In addition to conducting psychoanalytic psychotherapy, Kevin Volkan has worked in a wide variety of positions with many kinds of patients in situations that were not only non-psychoanalytic but also antithetical to psychoanalysis in general. Nevertheless, even in the presence of hostility toward psychoanalytic clinical approaches, he has found that psychoanalysis offered key insights and techniques that helped the people with whom he was working.

Kevin Volkan has written psychoanalytic books exploring drug addiction and schizophrenia, as well as numerous psychoanalytic articles examining demonic possession, dissociative disorders, hoarding, personality disorders, sexual fetishes, and also non-clinical applications of psychoanalysis to Buddhism, organizational psychology, and even reality television (K. Volkan, 1994a, 1994b, 2013a, 2013b, 2014, 2016, 2020a, 2020b, 2021a, 2021b; K. Volkan & V. D. Volkan, 2022). In addition to case histories, quantitative scientific studies inform his work.

This book tells the reader how the human mind works, illustrates psychoanalytic terms and concepts with case examples, describes how psychoanalytic psychotherapy is conducted, and compares psycho-analytic psychotherapy to psychoanalysis proper. Its aim is to improve psychoanalytic psychotherapists' professional identities as well as their approaches to their patients. The book explores psychotherapeutic approaches to individuals with various types of traumas and personality organizations. It is our sincere hope that this book will be of benefit to students of all therapeutic persuasions studying clinical psychology as well as members of the general public who are interested in exploring how the human mind works.

Terminology

We will use several terms to refer to those who practice psychoanalysis and psychoanalytic psychotherapy throughout this book. The two main terms are *psychoanalyst* (or *analyst*) and *psychoanalytic psychotherapist* (or *psychodynamic psychotherapist*). These terms are distinguishable, and a bit of explanation is in order.

A *psychoanalyst* is someone who has received advanced training at a psychoanalytic institute beyond his or her graduate degree. A psychoanalyst has had several years of coursework (five or more in some institutes), undergone psychoanalysis themselves as part of his or her training, and has completed several psychoanalytic cases under the supervision of an experienced psychoanalyst. Requirements vary depending on the specific institute and the institute's theoretical orientation; for example, some institutes require completion of a dissertation on a psychoanalytic subject. Some states in the USA, such as New York, license psychoanalysts while most others require that psychoanalysts already be licensed in a mental health profession. However, in most states, "psychoanalyst" is a term of art reserved for those who have official training, without which a person may not hold himself or herself out to the public as a psychoanalyst. In this book, the term "psychoanalyst" (unless specifically mentioned) will refer to Freudian and neo-Freudian analysts.

A *psychoanalytic psychotherapist* is someone who holds a graduate degree in a mental health field and is licensed to practice psychotherapy. This person has undergone a training program, either formal or informal, in psychoanalytic psychotherapy. Many psychoanalytic institutes now have such training programs. These programs generally require two or more years of coursework as well as experience being supervised by a psychoanalyst or advanced psychoanalytic psychotherapist for several clinical cases. One can also become a psychoanalytic psychotherapist by taking courses on one's own and then finding a psychoanalyst or psychoanalytic psychotherapist to provide supervision for several cases. While the term "psychotherapist" is a term of art reserved for people with a mental health practitioner's license, the term psychoanalytic psychotherapist is not. That means that anyone who is a licensed mental health care practitioner, who thinks they have enough training, can use this term. Like psychoanalysts, there are many different theoretical orientations among psychoanalytic psychotherapists. However, in this book the term *psychoanalytic psychotherapist* will refer to Freudian or neo-Freudian practitioners. These psychoanalytic psychotherapists typically will adhere to the same core principles as Freudian and neo-Freudian psychoanalysts.

A *psychodynamic psychotherapist* is someone who has had similar training as a psychoanalytic psychotherapist, but who may or may not adhere to certain core Freudian psychoanalytic principles. For instance, a psychodynamic psychotherapist may practice from an attachment perspective, where the type of relationship formed in early childhood is replayed out in adulthood. This type of practitioner may not believe in, or make use of, the understanding of drives in his or her practice. However, other psychodynamic psychotherapists may adhere to core Freudian concepts yet choose to call themselves psychodynamic psychotherapists rather than psychoanalytic psychotherapists because they may be concerned that the term "psychoanalytic" could cause confusion regarding whether the practitioner is an analyst. "Psychodynamic psychotherapist" is a loose term, and because of this we will use it sparingly in this book.

There are, of course, many exceptions to the above practitioner characterizations. For the purposes of this book, however, the above descriptions should provide some clarity regarding which type of practitioner we are describing.

Also, throughout this book we will frequently refer to psychoanalysts and psychoanalytic psychotherapists. The phrase *psychoanalysts and psychoanalytic psychotherapists* is, however, cumbersome. Therefore, we will use the term *psychoanalytic clinicians* when we refer to psychoanalysts and psychoanalytic psychotherapists collectively. We will also use the term *therapist* to refer more loosely to those who are mental health practitioners.

Another term than needs to be considered is the label we apply to those we work with therapeutically. This is a damned-if-you-do, damned-if-you-don't type of situation. Traditionally, physicians and psychologists have used the term *patient* as shorthand for those who suffer from psychopathology. Over the years, and especially after the human potential movement of the 1960s and 1970s, the word *patient* began to be seen as stigmatizing. This was especially true in an era where inhabitants of mental hospitals (i.e., patients) were part of a mental health system that often warehoused or abused people. The word patient also has strong connections to the medical profession. In the past, medical doctors had *patients*, while other mental healthcare workers had *clients*. The use of the word patient carried connotations of the medical doctor's authority, sometimes giving rise to a *built-in transference* (which we shall discuss in detail later). This situation has been muddied somewhat by the rise of doctoral level psychologists who *see patients* but also *have clients*. The profession of clinical psychology has for much of its history been excluded from medical guild status. Nowhere has this been truer than in American Freudian psychoanalysis, which has only wholesale opened psychoanalytic training to non-MDs since the late 1980s, and only under the injunction of multiple lawsuits (Simons, 2003). Nowadays, this situation seems to have resolved itself. Non-MDs are welcome to train at psychoanalytic institutes all across the United States and typically outnumber their MD colleagues (Katz et al., 2012).

Under the influence of practitioners such as Carl Rogers, psychotherapists of all types began addressing their patients as "clients." The term "client" was seen as less stigmatizing and perhaps minimized the idea that people were suffering from psychopathology. However, the word "client" also carries certain connotations. It implies a commercial relationship between a provider and a consumer. Fuller Torrey (2011) writes that the word "client" carries with it the idea that the person is a voluntary customer of legal or financial services. As Carlos Sluzki (2000) tells us, any relationship to consumerism, "... carries with it the assumption that there is an implicitly dangerous, exploitative relationship between a naive consumer, who needs protection by a benign advocate against a conniving exploiter" (p. 348).

Sluzki goes on to explain that the word *client* derives from the Latin *cluere*, which means to listen. The connotation is that a client is someone who listens to advice. Psychoanalysis and psychoanalytic psychotherapy, the subjects of this book, should not involve dispensing advice, and therefore the word client makes us uncomfortable.

The word *patient* on the other hand, according to Sluzki, derives from the Latin *pati*, which mean to suffer. "Other associations of the word 'patient' or 'patience' lead us to the sets enduring/stoical; serene/placid, and tenacious/unremitting" (p. 351). Here, we feel we can find more concordance with psychoanalytic clinical reality.

Pamela Hartzband and Jerome Groopman from Harvard are concerned that newer terminology for patients, such as consumer or client, is being driven by the industrialization and commercialization of medical care where hospitals are run like factories. They warn that good medical care takes time and that there are multiple paths to treatment (Hartzband & Groopman, 2011, 2016). This view is also consonant with psychoanalytic clinical practice where the course of treatment is somewhat unpredictable, and the clinician needs to improvise to some degree.

A survey of physicians and psychologists conducted by Ahsan Naseem and his colleagues (Naseem et al., 2001) indicates that both physicians and psychologists preferred to refer to those seeking their help as patients, though medical doctors preferred the use of last names while psychologists preferred first names. It seems that people using psychiatric clinics also prefer the term patient. A survey in the UK showed that 77% of people attending a psychiatric clinic preferred to be referred to as patients rather than clients. There were also no subgroups that preferred the word client (Ritchie et al., 2000). However, in more mixed settings that emphasize the role of the "consumer" of mental health services, the words consumer and client were preferred over the word patient (Lloyd et al., 2001).

There is no perfect term to describe those with whom we work. Given the above thoughts, however, we are more comfortable using the term patient in this book.

CHAPTER 1

Psychoanalysis and psychoanalytic psychotherapy: Five therapeutic principles

There is a great deal of confusion among clinicians and members of the public about psychoanalysis proper and psychoanalytic psychotherapy. This is true even among the practitioners of these methods. One of the reasons for this is the sheer number of types of psychoanalysis and psychoanalytic psychotherapies that are currently practiced around the world. Many of these are similar and others are divergent. It would be impossible in a short book such as this one to list all of these or to review all the characteristics of each. Instead, we will present a sort of hypothetical median to define what is meant by Freudian-derived psychoanalysis and psychoanalytic psychotherapy based on the authors' experiences and perception of the field. While we present what we consider to be those theories and techniques most often encompassed by Freudian and neo-Freudian psychoanalytic clinicians, we also acknowledge (and from time to time draw upon) many different schools of thought. These schools of practice and thought use similar terms but can diverge widely from what we are stating as a sort of "standard." Perhaps this is a limitation of our work. But it is also a strength in that we are attempting to establish core psychoanalytic ideas while explaining the different ways these can manifest clinically.

Let us go back to Sigmund Freud and the early times of psychoanalysis. Sigmund Freud (1919a) and Edward Glover (1931) wrote about the differences between psychoanalysis and psychoanalytic psychotherapy and viewed psychoanalytic psychotherapy largely as a work of suggestions. Edward Bibring (1954) mentioned five therapeutic principles in comparing psychotherapies with psychoanalysis. These principles are suggestion, abreaction, manipulation, clarification, and interpretation.

1. *Suggestion* refers to the therapist's inducing various mental processes in his or her patient independently of—or to the exclusion of—the patient's rational or critical thinking. For example, the psychotherapist helps a patient to try a different response to a certain situation.

2. *Abreaction* describes an emotional discharge, an emotional reliving. For example, let us refer to a male patient who had an unloving mother. Because of this childhood experience, he kept an emotional distance from his wife, another woman, during adulthood. During his psychotherapy, this man spoke of his wife's death two years prior to his starting his treatment. He described in detail, without exhibiting any emotions, how his wife died after most of her skin was burned in a house on fire. One day, while referring to the death of his wife, the patient suddenly started crying, hitting his head with his hands, and screaming—openly expressing various emotions such as sadness, anger, and guilt and thus having an abreaction experience.

   In the early days of psychoanalysis, abreaction was considered a curative process. Bibring (1954) stated that abreaction as a curative principle is, to a certain degree, maintained. But the value of the emotional discharge should be considered only in combination with other therapeutic principles.

3. *Manipulation* is used to produce in the patient a favorable attitude toward the treatment situation and exposing the patient to a "new" experience with which the patient had not previously been acquainted or had not experienced since childhood. Bibring (1954) describes the patient embarking on treatment at the instance of some authoritarian influence. When the therapist convinces this patient that it is up to him or her whether or

not to discuss his or her problems in their sessions, the therapist reestablishes the patient's freedom of choice. One benefit of this is that the patient then feels that he or she is expected to act on his or her own responsibility.

Bibring tells us that suggestion, abreaction, and manipulation do not give the patient self-understanding. Instead, the remaining two therapeutic principles, clarification and interpretation, accomplish this.

4. *Clarification* does not expose unconscious material but material that simply escapes the patient's attention and is more or less easily recognized by him or her when his or her attention is directed to it. Bibring (1954) writes that clarification "refers to those techniques and therapeutic processes that assist the patient to reach a higher degree of self-awareness, clarity and differentiation of self-observation that makes adequate verbalization possible" (p. 755).

5. *Interpretation* refers to the uncovering of unconscious material; it is a prolonged process rather than a single act. Insight brought about by interpretation differs from that effected by clarification. Clarification helps the patient to achieve greater objectivity whereas interpretation "leads to the reactivation of painful tendencies, memories and conflicts" (Bibring, 1954, p. 758).

When Edward Bibring wrote his paper in 1954, insight through interpretation was considered the principal agent of change. Salman Akhtar (2009) referred to ideas of psychoanalysts expressed in the 1980s and 1990s and stated that similarities between psychoanalysis and psychoanalytic psychotherapy are accepted if both types of work with patients focus on exploring unconscious issues, the importance of childhood experiences, transference, and countertransference (also see: Gill, 1994; Kernberg, 1984a; Pine, 1997).

Transference and countertransference

Briefly, the term transference refers to a patient's experiencing the psychoanalyst's image as an image or images of other important individuals in his or her life, especially during the patient's childhood. This includes parents, other caregivers, siblings, and individuals involved with traumatic events in the patient's life. The term countertransference is used when we refer to a psychoanalytic clinician's own feelings and attitudes influenced by his or her earlier relations with important others now directed toward a patient.

Obviously, the contrast between a psychoanalyst sitting behind a patient who lies on the psychoanalytic couch four or five times a week and a psychoanalytic psychotherapist meeting with a patient face-to-face once or twice a week leads to significant differences between the two types of treatment. The intensity of the development and exploration of unconscious issues, the understanding of the importance of the role of childhood experiences in forming the patient's symptoms and personality characteristics, and the therapeutic roles of transference and countertransference will be different.

Differences between psychoanalysis and psychoanalytic psychotherapy

In general, the aim of psychoanalytic psychotherapy is to help people to deal with psychologically troublesome events, as well as alleviate symptoms that were troubling enough to cause someone to seek treatment. Both these events and symptoms have an origin in the unconscious. The aim of psychoanalysis is deeper: a successful psychoanalytic process leads to making positive structural modifications in the analysand's mind and mental functions. However, going through a long-term psychoanalytic psychotherapy may also help patients to develop more adaptive and less anxiety-provoking ways to live. Akhtar (2009) states: "In essence, all analyses include interventions that are essentially psychotherapeutic, and all significant psychotherapies done by an analyst have elements of psychoanalysis. It is a continuum of dimensions that one is dealing with here, and not a cubicle of categories" (p. 231).

We can summarize these ideas by saying that psychoanalysis enables fundamental changes in the patient's personality, while psychoanalytic psychotherapy helps the patient adapt his or her personality to his or her life circumstances. While personality change may result from psychoanalytic psychotherapy, it does not generally result in as far-reaching fundamental personality change as what can be achieved in psychoanalysis.

There are also psychotherapists who have not gone through a personal analysis and formal psychoanalytic training. Throughout four decades, V. D. Volkan has supervised the therapeutic work of more than twenty such psychiatrists, psychologists, and social workers in the United States and other countries. To a lesser extent, K. Volkan has supervised several psychoanalytic psychotherapists as well as guiding them through their doctoral and postdoctoral training. We have been impressed by the ability of most of these psychoanalytic psychotherapists to benefit from supervision and the application of psychoanalytic concepts to successfully treat their patients. Nevertheless, change in an individual's personality generally occurs in a more limited way in psychoanalytic psychotherapy when compared to individuals who go through psychoanalysis.

The caveat here is that the difference between psychotherapy and analysis may be one of time and exposure. Brief psychodynamic therapies may be more limited, focused as they are on symptom reduction rather than personality change. But a long, intensive psychoanalytic therapy may achieve goals similar to those achieved after analysis. Likewise, psychoanalytic therapy is less standardized and applied in many different ways. Changes in the mind of an individual in psychoanalytic psychotherapy are likely more dependent on who is doing the therapy and the types of theory and techniques of psychoanalysis the therapist employs.

There is a gray area between psychoanalysis and psychoanalytic psychotherapy. It is perhaps helpful to think of these as ends of a therapeutic spectrum. While psychoanalysis is the more in-depth end of the therapeutic spectrum, it is not always the superior approach. This will depend on the needs of the patient and what modality is best for each patient's unique situation and constellation of pathology.

Starting when Sigmund Freud was alive, there have been different "schools" of psychoanalysis. For example, during Freud's time some psychoanalysts were followers of Carl Jung. Now psychoanalysts are known as followers of classical, interpersonal, or relational psychoanalysis or are labeled as ego psychologists, self-psychologists, Freudian, Jungian, Kleinian, Bionian, Fairbairnian, Winnicottian, Lacanian, and so on. Increased variety of therapeutic approaches—all of which are called "psychoanalytic"—creates complexity in clinical judgments. In this book we try not to hide behind a specific school of psychoanalysis.

Instead, we will describe and examine key theoretical and technical psychoanalytic concepts and terms going back to Freud's and/or early psychoanalysts' descriptions and then add newer related findings. We will compare present-day conceptions about the main processes for making changes in a person's mind during psychoanalysis to these foundational concepts and terms. Knowledge about these concepts and terms—both foundational and present-day—is essential to conduct psychoanalytically informed psychotherapy. Besides illustrating these concepts and terms with case vignettes, we will include what we consider as important references to them.

"One psychoanalysis or many?"

The existence of different schools in psychoanalysis has created an increasing variety of therapeutic approaches. This so-called pluralism in psychoanalysis was brought to our attention in 1988 when then president of the International Psychoanalytical Association Robert Wallerstein posed the question, "One psychoanalysis or many?" (Wallerstein, 1988). The diverse theoretical and technical considerations within the psychoanalytic circles of today give us a clear answer.

The primary change, as André Green (2000) stated, has been the focus on the role of the object, such as a child's mother, and the relationship between instinctual drive and object, the latter being unduly neglected in classical Freudian theory. As a response to the growth of pluralism, some analysts, notably Leo Rangell (2000), proposed a united and composite theory of psychoanalysis that is to be distinguished from non-psychoanalytic theories of mental life. But the growth of pluralism also brought forth attempts that can be seen as "throwing the baby out with the bathwater," and that have created unnecessary and destructive competition. Green (2000) referred to a pointless struggle for supremacy between those who focus on the intrapsychic and those who follow intersubjective processes in psychoanalysis, since both processes play a part in any analytic treatment.

We agree with Tomas Böhm (2002), who stated that different ways of listening to the patient and different styles of handling clinical material began to put analysts in completely different professions. What is psychoanalytic treatment? Who is a psychoanalyst? Otto Kernberg's (2001) overview of psychoanalytic technique (according to various schools of thought) was an attempt to answer these questions.

Some essential theoretical as well as technical concepts have been questioned in the culture of pluralism. For example, Peter Fonagy (1999) challenged Sigmund Freud's (1914d) belief that the theory of repression is the cornerstone on which the whole structure of psychoanalysis rests. Fonagy stated that psychoanalysts should avoid digging in the buried past and bringing it to light. He stated that "the archeological metaphor" (p. 220) should not be a focus for the psychoanalytic technique; instead, psychoanalysts should rely exclusively on the current transference. According to him, the only way psychoanalysts could know "what goes on in our patients' minds, what might have happened to them, is how they are with us in the transference" (p. 217). While Fonagy's reference to the role of transference in treating an individual is correct, we also agree with Harold Blum (2003), who strongly questioned Fonagy's assertion. Blum stated: "Without the patient's life story, including education, family and culture, as well as character, the transference cannot be fully understood and vice versa" (p. 498).

The scope of psychoanalysis and psychoanalytic psychotherapy

In 1953, some well-known psychoanalysts discussed the "widening scope of psychoanalysis" (A. Freud, 1954; Jacobson, 1954; Stone, 1954; Weigert, 1954). During this discussion, Anna Freud said:

> If all the skill, knowledge and pioneering effort which was spent on widening the scope of application of psychoanalysis had been employed instead on intensifying and improving our technique in the original field, I cannot help but feel that, by now, we would find the treatment of the common neuroses child's play, instead of struggling with their technical problems as we have continued to do. How do analysts decide if they are given the choice between returning to health half a dozen young people with good prospects in life but disturbed in their enjoyment and efficiency by comparatively mild neuroses, or to devote the same time, trouble, and effort to one single borderline case, who may or may not be saved from spending the rest of his life in an institution? Personally, I can

feel the pull in both directions, perhaps with a bias toward the former task; as a body, the [American] Psychoanalytic Association has inclined in recent years toward the latter. (A. Freud, 1954, pp. 610–611)

Today patients with so-called narcissistic and borderline personality disorders fill psychoanalysts' and psychoanalytic therapists' offices. Most psychotherapists have not received proper training and experience to successfully treat these kinds of patients. Also, these patients are notoriously difficult to treat in psychotherapy; this serves as a disincentive for psychotherapists to work with these kinds of patients.

Much the same is true for people suffering from psychoses. Although people suffering from psychoses are not filling psychotherapists' offices, the predominant treatment—medication—is not effective at alleviating psychosis, but serves only to reduce its symptoms. This can easily be seen in the large numbers of homeless mentally ill people populating most major cities in the United States. For all practical purposes, the psychoanalytic treatment of people suffering from psychosis that was practiced in the 1960s and 1970s has almost disappeared in the United States. Nevertheless, newer research findings ranging from epigenetics to social cognition give an indication that psychotherapeutic treatment, and specifically psychoanalytic treatment, may be effective in treating some cases of psychosis (K. Volkan & V. D. Volkan, 2022).

Fortunately, psychoanalysis and psychoanalytic psychotherapy have matured to the point where the full spectrum of mental disorders can be successfully treated. In addition to treating people with neuroses, psychoanalysis and psychoanalytic psychotherapy are being used to treat people suffering from personality disorders (Kernberg, 1975, 1984a; V. D. Volkan, 1987) and schizophrenia (K. Volkan & V. D. Volkan, 2022). Psychoanalysis and psychoanalytic psychotherapy have also moved beyond the therapy hour and are useful in examining business organizations (e.g., Kernberg, 1984b; K. Volkan, 1994a) and the psychology of large groups and pathological leaders (K. Volkan, 2021a; V. D. Volkan, 2018, 2020), as well as resolving international conflicts (V. D. Volkan, 1988, 2006b, 2013). Psychoanalytic concepts have also been used to understand religions and popular culture (K. Volkan, 2013a, 2013b, 2014).

Psychiatry, psychotherapy, and psychoanalysis

Recent studies show that the number of people, overall, seeking psychotherapy from a psychiatrist in the United States has declined. A study by Daniel Tadmon and Mark Olfson published in *The American Journal of Psychiatry* (2022) illustrates that the percentage of visits to a psychiatrist involving psychotherapy in the United States dropped more than 50% between 1996 and 2016. Another study by James Rim and his colleagues (Rim et al., 2020) showed that 74% of psychiatric residency programs do not include psychotherapy training and that most of these programs do not intend to add this type of training in the future. Mark Moran (2022) states that this "public health crisis [is] driven by an insurance industry that disincentivizes treatment aimed at recovery by the most highly trained practitioners" (p. 1).

That most psychiatrists no longer practice psychotherapy makes sense from a purely monetary point of view. Medication consultation is far more lucrative than practicing psychotherapy. As of this writing, a psychiatrist in the United States can see four patients in an hour, billing in the vicinity of $350–$500 per patient or $1400–$2000 per hour. Much of this cost will be covered by the patient's health insurance. A psychiatrist seeing a patient for a fifty-minute session of psychoanalysis or psychotherapy will bill between $250 and $500 an hour, and most of this cost will not be covered by insurance, at least after the first few sessions. It is no wonder that new psychiatrists, who are often saddled with large school loan debts, choose not to seek expertise in psychoanalysis or psychotherapy.

Additionally, there is a shortage of psychiatrists in the United States, with few medical students choosing psychiatry as a specialty. On the other hand, the number of doctoral-level psychologists is stable, with the number of female and racial minority psychologists on the rise (L. Lin et al., 2015). While most of these psychologists will not become psychoanalytic clinicians, some will, and so these numbers will increase. Clearly, the future of psychoanalysis and psychoanalytic psychotherapy will be in the hands of doctoral-level psychologists, and to some degree master's degree-level practitioners. The era of psychoanalysis being predominantly performed by medical doctors is over in the United States. A recent experience illustrates this change. We were at a lecture in a large city at a psychoanalytic institute where Vamık Volkan was giving a talk. On one side of the room, the psychoanalysts were gathered. This was a gray-haired bunch, mostly men over sixty with MD degrees. On the other side of the room, the psychoanalytic psychotherapists were gathered. By and large, these were young women in their thirties with doctorates in psychology. The contrast was stark.

In writing this book, we kept the above information in mind. We want to provide a source of uncomplicated information about psychoanalytic concepts, illustrated by various case histories drawn from psychoanalysis and psychoanalytic psychotherapy. This will be useful not only to those training in psychoanalysis proper and psychoanalytic psychotherapy, but also to interested clinicians who practice other types of psychotherapy.

CHAPTER 2

Id, ego, superego

S ince the aim of psychoanalysis as well as psychoanalytic psychotherapy is to make positive changes in an individual mind, we
start this chapter by describing Sigmund Freud's (1923b, 1933a,
1940a) structural model of mind. We then refer to newer psychoanalytic theories and findings about how a child's mind develops. Adding
new findings to, and making some modifications of, Freud's thinking
enriches psychoanalytic theories and clinical work.

The id—Eros and Thanatos

Sigmund Freud's structural model divides the mind into three sections:
id, ego, and superego. Freud stated that the id is present at birth and
is a container of inherited sexual and aggressive instincts or drives.
The id has two aspects: Eros and Thanatos. The aim of Eros is to create
and preserve ever-greater unities. The aim of Thanatos is to break down
and destroy connections.

Some psychoanalytic theorists and practitioners from the more relational schools now believe these instincts lack clinical utility. But these
drives are important. Freud (1914c) is clear about this when he states
"… I should like at this point expressly to admit that the hypothesis

of separate ego-instincts and sexual instincts (that is to say, the libido theory) rests scarcely at all upon a psychological basis, but derives its principal support from biology" (p. 144). The reason drives exist is to help us survive. In fact, Eros and Thanatos can be observed in all animals—and perhaps all living creatures. Eros is fundamentally a drive to procreate, eat, and excrete—all of which are necessary for survival. Evolution for the most part has rendered these as pleasurable activities. These survival activities stimulate the brain's circuitry such that we experience pleasure. If something is pleasurable, we seek to repeat it.

Thanatos, on the other hand, can be understood simply as a capacity for aggression. If you attack and corner an animal, it will fight back. Animals will attack and kill other animals for food. Without this kind of aggressive drive, animals will not be able to survive and make more of themselves. Therefore, there is strong evolutionary pressure in most animals to defend themselves and/or be able to kill for their dinner.

The circuitries for both Eros and Thanatos are wired into our brains. They are important in that they tie psychoanalysis to our biology in a profound way. These drives are as old as the emergence of life on planet Earth. Eros and Thanatos, making up the id, are the engines of the structure of our minds, as well as the origins of our thoughts, behaviors, and emotions.

All the id's activities are unconscious. They are governed by so-called "primary process," in which there is no recognition of good and bad or yes and no. For humans there is greater survival value (or what evolutionary biologists term "fitness") if there is some regulation of the id. Humans have evolved patterns of behavior and lifestyles that require cooperation. For this to occur, our pleasurable and aggressive passions must be channeled. This is accomplished by the ego.

The ego

In 1933, Freud reminded us that where the id was, there the ego shall be. Because of the influence of the real external world, a part of the id, its "cortical layer," undergoes a change and evolves as ego. "The ego represents what may be called reason and common sense, in contrast to the id, which contains passions" (Freud, 1923b, p. 25). The ego has both conscious and unconscious parts and uses rationality, the so-called "secondary process," and deals with realities of the external world, safety, and timing. Libido (the emotional and psychic energy associated with Eros and Thanatos) is stored in the ego. Freud (1940a) described this situation as "primary narcissism." Primary narcissism changes when the ego starts to cathect (i.e., connect to) images of objects (usually primary caregivers) with libido. This transforms narcissistic libido into object libido. Freud also explained that the most prominent areas of the body from which the libido arises are oral, anal, and phallic zones.

The superego

Another important psychic structure is the superego. The super-ego carries our sense of morality and functions as our conscience. In normal individuals, the superego is impartial; however, for neurotic people, Freud (1926e) says,

> Their super-ego still confronts their ego as a strict father confronts a child; and their morality operates in a primitive fashion in that the ego gets itself punished by the super-ego. Illness is employed as an instrument for this "self-punishment", and neurotics have to behave as though they were governed by a sense of guilt which, to be satisfied, needs to be punished by illness. (p. 223)

Freud wrote that the superego develops "from an identification with the father taken as a model" (Freud, 1923b, p. 54). Therefore, we can imagine the superego as an inner voice, an older caretaker's injunctions and prohibitions, an inner authority or judge. Hence the superego is also a source of internal guilt.

The superego contains the ego ideal, which Freud (1914c; 1923b) tells us is derived from a representation of our relationship with our parents, who stand in for our higher and best selves when we are children. Where the ego represents the external world, the superego represents the internal world, and this leads to conflicts between the ego and the superego. This is related to the Oedipus complex (to be discussed later). The superego contains the fear of conscience. The superior being (father) represents the ego ideal. However, because of the Oedipus complex, he also threatens castration, and, "... this dread of castration is probably the nucleus round which the subsequent fear of conscience has gathered; it is this dread that persists as the fear of conscience" (p. 57).

The development of the superego also confers fitness to humans, allowing for more successful social interactions and channeling of the id (Freud, 1914c).

The relationship between id, ego, and superego

The id and superego have one thing in common: both represent the influences of the past. The id represents the influence of heredity, and the superego represents the influence of what was assimilated from other individuals. The ego is determined by the person's own experiences (Freud, 1940a).

Freud (1923b) described the relationship between the id and the ego as that between a horse and its rider. The horse represents the id, and the rider stands for the ego. In making this analogy, Freud did not refer to the superego. Let us put a fence around the location where the horse and the rider are present and consider this fence as the superego, restricting the area where the rider and horse travel.

The aim of psychoanalytic therapy—and in more depth, psychoanalysis—is to help the rider understand the nature of his or her horse's impulses better and develop new skills (new ego functions) to make riding the horse smoother, less dangerous, more enjoyable, and more adaptive. Also, psychoanalysis and psychoanalytic therapy allow the rider to make changes in the location of the fence, allowing the horseback rides to take place in a larger and safer arena. This reflects taming the superego's restrictions as well making its function more realistic.

CHAPTER 3

Psychotherapeutic identity, confidentiality, and psychotherapist disclosure

L et us imagine an adult man who starts having pain around his belly button. Then the pain progresses to the lower right abdomen or pelvis. He also experiences fever and nausea. In other words, this person has symptoms of appendicitis. He goes to see a surgeon, who, besides his own skills achieved through observing and assisting experienced surgeons' work, also uses a surgical knife, and now, with the advancement of technology, a laparoscopic instrument. The surgeon knows that the surgical knife or another instrument is sterilized before cutting or entering into the skin of the patient to remove the appendix. He or she has external tools.

When an individual has emotional problems, he or she may seek help from a psychotherapist. Some psychotherapists prescribe medications as well as provide opinions and suggestions. They utilize medications and advice as tools for treatment. Psychoanalytic clinicians, in addition to knowledge they have received about psychoanalytic and psycho-therapeutic concepts, utilize their therapeutic identities as "therapeutic instruments" (Olinick, 1980).

The term identity refers to an individual's inner working model—this person, not an outsider, senses and experiences it. Every person has an individual identity, "a persistent sameness within oneself" as well as "a persistent sharing of some kind of essential character with others" (Erikson, 1956, p. 57). Psychoanalytic clinicians also develop a "therapeutic identity" during their training and while receiving supervision. They hold on to this identity while working with their patients.

Due to different factors, such as the nature of personality organization, education, training, supervision, and the frequency of therapeutic sessions, psychoanalytic clinicians' effectiveness varies when they first start clinical practice. As they become more experienced, however, these professionals will develop a strong therapeutic identity that will be their key therapeutic instrument, allowing them to successfully treat those who come to them for help.

Patient confidentiality

In his or her clinical office, a psychoanalytic therapist holds on to his or her therapeutic identity and knows that listening to, and talking with, a patient is unlike any other social relationship. When a person seeks treatment, a psychoanalytic clinician instructs the patient to feel free to say whatever comes into his or her mind and adds that whatever the patient says will stay between them. This is a direct sharing of a crucial aspect of the psychoanalytic clinician's therapeutic identity with the patient; the clinician is a person who will respect and protect confidentiality. The clinician will not share or discuss what he or she hears from the patient outside the clinical office. If the therapist is receiving supervision, we know that the supervisor also possesses a therapeutic identity and will keep information about the patient confidential. As in this book, and while making professional presentations, we do tell some patients' stories, but we do so in a way that the true identity of each patient remains hidden. In a perfect world, confidentiality would remain between the clinician and the patient. However, over the years, the limits of confidentiality have necessarily been modified.

On October 27, 1969, Tatiana Tarasoff was killed by her ex-boyfriend Prosenjit Poddar, who was also a University of California graduate student. During his seventh psychotherapy session at the university counseling center with psychologist Lawrence Moore, Poddar revealed that he was going to kill Tarasoff. Moore consulted with the head of psychiatry and it was agreed that he should contact the police about the threat. Moore called and sent a letter to the campus police outlining his view that Poddar was paranoid and a credible threat to Tarasoff. The police contacted Poddar but did not hold him for observation. Instead, they told him to stay away from Tarasoff. When Dr. Moore's supervisor Harvey Powelson found out that he had contacted the police about Poddar, he directed the police to return Moore's warning letter, and told Moore to destroy all clinical records of the case and not place Poddar on a seventy-two hour hold in a treatment facility. At no point was Tatiana Tarasoff informed that her ex-boyfriend had threatened to kill her.

Sadly, two months later, Poddar went to Tarasoff's house, shot her with a pellet gun and then brutally stabbed her to death with a large butcher knife. He then called the police and turned himself in. Poddar was convicted of second-degree murder; however, the conviction was overturned on a technicality and he was deported to India.

Tarasoff's parents sued the clinicians, the police, and the university for negligence in not preventing their daughter's death. They initially lost their case, but it was taken on appeal to the California Supreme Court, which ruled in 1976 that through the actions of its employees the university was negligent in Tarasoff's death by not exercising a reasonable duty to warn the victim. This resulted in the so-called Tarasoff rule, whereby clinicians who have a patient that demonstrates they are a danger to others have an obligation to use reasonable care to protect the intended victim(s) against that danger (Lipson & Mills, 1998). In 1985, the California legislature codified and somewhat narrowed the Tarasoff rule, such that a psychotherapist has a duty to warn and take steps to protect an intended victim only if the therapist actually believes or predicts that the patient poses a serious risk of inflicting serious bodily injury upon a reasonably identifiable victim or victims.

This case had a great deal of impact around the United States, with many states creating similar rules that include the breach of psychotherapeutic confidentiality. It is now important for psychoanalytic clinicians to understand the "duty to warn" rules where they practice as there is considerable variation among these in the United States (Johnson et al., 2014).

On June 27, 1991, in Illinois, United States, a female police officer, Mary Lou Redmond, shot and killed Ricky Allen, who was about to stab a man with a knife he was carrying. After Ricky Allen died, a representative of his estate, Carrie Jaffe, filed a suit claiming that Redmond used excessive force. Jaffe also learned that Redmond had sought therapeutic help from a social worker and demanded that this psychotherapist's notes be available to Allen's estate attorneys during the police officer's cross-examination at trial. This event resulted in the United States Supreme Court asserting that confidentiality in psychotherapy may take precedence over other societal goals. In its 1996 ruling, the Court interpreted the Federal Rules of Evidence to include a psychotherapist–patient privilege. This ruling, however, "applied only to whether a patient or therapist could be compelled to disclose the content of therapy sessions in the course of a civil proceeding. Lower courts have begun to consider application of privilege in criminal cases, but this has not yet been established" (Dewald & Clark, 2001, p. 22). Additional exceptions to the confidentiality of psychotherapy are recognized by various jurisdictions, for example, where there is a reasonable suspicion of child abuse or elder adult physical abuse; where there is a reasonable suspicion that a patient may present a danger of violence to others; and where there is a reasonable suspicion that a patient is likely to harm themself unless protective measures are taken. Moreover, a patient may also be required to waive the privilege, for example, if he or she chooses to put his or her mental state at issue in a civil case (where he or she seeks compensation for emotional distress) or a criminal case (where he or she raises an insanity defense).

As a result of the legal landscape governing the therapeutic privilege and its exceptions, many mental health practitioners have modified the way in which they take and keep clinical notes. Some psychotherapists, knowing that the confidentiality of their notes could be breached, have chosen to record a bare minimum of information in an official clinical record—usually a diagnosis, therapeutic techniques employed, and a statement about the patient's progress. This is a problem when complete detailed note-taking is clearly a better practice. This is especially true for psychoanalytic clinicians. Jon Mills from Canada has proposed a separation of process notes from an official clinical record with the idea that only the official clinical record would be shared with third parties, while the process notes would be privileged and kept confidential. However, most court systems do not recognize this separation, meaning that all records may be subject to disclosure (Mills, 2015). This is clearly an area where psychotherapists of all types should work for reform.

Regardless of the type of psychotherapy, breaking a patient's confidentiality will have a serious impact on the course of treatment. In psychoanalysis and psychoanalytic psychotherapy, however, there is a further problem in that therapeutic neutrality and abstinence are also compromised. We will cover these important topics further below. What is important to know is that there may be circumstances when the psychoanalytic clinician will be required to break confidentiality, either because the patient threatens harm to others or to themselves. It is usually wise to discuss or provide information to patients about the limits of confidentiality. Patients need to be aware of what happens if the analyst or therapist learns or senses that the patient is involved or may be involved in a legal issue. This should be discussed before beginning treatment. Otherwise, if a situation arises where confidentiality must be breached, we might scare the patient and undermine his or her trust in the therapeutic process. In a way, the limits of confidentiality are a container around the therapeutic encounter reminding the patient that they should refrain from acting out during the course of treatment.

Psychotherapist disclosure

A psychoanalytic psychotherapist pays serious attention to keeping details of his or her personal life away from his or her patients. We will illustrate the concept of transference in detail later in this book. Here, we are focusing on how a psychoanalytic therapist needs confidentiality about his or her personal life.

Vamık Volkan had his psychiatric residency from 1958 to 1962 at the Department of Psychiatry, University of North Carolina, in Chapel Hill, North Carolina. After working at a hospital in North Carolina for two more years, he moved to Virginia and started his academic life at the University of Virginia in Charlottesville, Virginia. At this time, in the late 1960s, he became a psychoanalyst. During those years, since English was not his original language, his patients would notice his accent right away. Vamık Volkan was born to Turkish parents on the Mediterranean island of Cyprus. He came to the United States in early 1957 as a new graduate of a medical school in Turkey. Some of his patients would ask about his ethnic background. He would respond by telling them, "Let us wait to see what kinds of thoughts you will have about my background as we continue working together." During the 1950s and 1960s, it was rather easy to keep personal history away from patients. Incredible developments in communication technology during the last few decades now make it almost impossible to "hide" information about oneself. Our advice to younger psychoanalytic clinicians is to be careful not to make available detailed personal stories about themselves that can be read or watched on computers and other similar devices.

Again, psychoanalytic clinicians have perhaps a greater burden in keeping their private lives inaccessible to their patients since their therapeutic technique relies on neutrality and abstinence. Greta Kaluzeviciute (2020), in her recent writing on social media and its impact on therapeutic relationships, reports that non-psychoanalytic psychotherapists tend toward greater breaches in their privacy due to having less inhibition about their online presence. This may be because therapist non-disclosure plays a lesser role in, or is not part of, their therapeutic technique. Psychotherapy systems generally frown upon therapists disclosing much information about themselves. However, this is something that is also highly variable. We have seen therapists who routinely self-disclose as an aspect of their technique. Kevin Volkan knew a therapist who would interrupt his patient's narrative and tell the patient all about his own problems. The idea was that this would distract the patient from his or her own problems! It is questionable whether this practice should even be called psychotherapy, and it borders on being unethical.

Advice-giving, which is commonly seen in the counseling profession and in some non-psychoanalytically-derived psychotherapies, is a close cousin to therapist self-disclosure. This is because the nature of the advice reveals a lot about the therapist. This is another reason, besides contaminating the transference, that psychoanalytic clinicians should avoid advice-giving. Kevin Volkan had a psychoanalyst as a clinical supervisor and mentor who had himself been in analysis for a long time. When asked about advice-giving, the supervisor reported that his analyst had only given him six words of advice in eight years of five-days-a-week analysis. One day near the end of his analysis, the supervisor was free-associating on the couch and said something about needing a new car. The next time there was a pause in his narrative, the supervisor's analyst quietly said, "I heard Hondas are good cars." That was the only advice the supervisor received in over 2000 hours of psychoanalysis.

Psychoanalytic clinicians who highly value non-disclosure tend to have less of an online presence, but this leads to its own issues. Patients of psychoanalytic practitioners may seek to recreate an online presence for their therapists and/or their therapeutic situation. In the absence of online information, some patients may create virtual manifestations of their therapist and their therapeutic situation leading to virtual versions of resistance and defense.

How does the psychoanalytic psychotherapist deal with this? Both authors of this book have appeared in national and international television media, as well as in films, podcasts, and other public forums. Sometimes our patients have viewed or heard these appearances and have learned something of our private lives. We have found that when this occurs, it is best not to deny the information that has been revealed but to be curious about how it has affected the patient. For instance, when a patient saw one of us on television and remarked that she hadn't realized that her therapist taught at a certain institution, the response was to ask why the patient found this interesting. We do not confirm or deny the information, but instead explore what it means to the patient. This sometimes leads to fruitful discussions that can reveal a good deal about the patient's transference to the clinician. It is important in such instances for the psychoanalytic clinician to pay close attention to his or her countertransference and counterresponses. At times, it may also be necessary to set boundaries. This may become imperative with patients who already have trouble with boundaries, such as those suffering from personality disorders.

Kevin Volkan was working with a patient who suffered from borderline personality disorder who found out that he lived in a city by the ocean. This patient then started to relate fantasies about visiting the city and the beach. These fantasies escalated to trying to find out where her therapist lived and showing up at his house. It was necessary to tell this patient that if she carried out her fantasy it would not be possible to remain as her psychotherapist and to help her get better. With this patient, it was especially important to set boundaries since she employed a primitive splitting defense where she would sometimes idealize and love the psychotherapist and other times devalue and be aggressive toward him. As Otto Kernberg (1975) states,

> At times the psychotherapist has to spell out certain conditions which the patient must meet in order for outpatient psycho-analytic psychotherapy to proceed … prohibiting patients from damaging or destroying objects in the psychotherapist's office, and prohibiting patients from actively trying to control the psycho-therapist's life outside the treatment hours all represent, it seems to me, occasionally necessary efforts on the part of the psychother-apist to protect a technically neutral treatment atmosphere … (pp. 189–190)

The internet and social media have made this much more difficult, and it may be that psychoanalytic technique will need to be adapted to our new therapeutic reality.

Given the rise of the internet and social media, it seems that psychoanalytic training for both analysts and therapists does need to be updated. Now that patients can easily find information about their therapists, psychoanalytic training may need to be enhanced with regards to the interrelated concepts of therapeutic identity, neutrality, and countertransference. It is possible to envision a course for psycho-analytic and psychotherapy trainees focused specifically on therapeu-tic identity. This course would address the maintenance of therapeutic identity in the face of patients having knowledge of the therapist's private life. Patients having this information are more likely to elicit a countertransference reaction from the therapist, so more training on dealing with countertransference should be included. The knowl-edge gained in this course would be reinforced by the exercise of *in vivo* skills.

Psychotherapeutic supervision could be enhanced by including additional practice dealing with the loss of psychotherapist privacy and countertransference reactions. This would be somewhere between standard supervision and the clinician's own therapy. During these sessions, the trainee could learn to deal with countertransference related to the involuntary disclosure of his or her personal information. For instance, these sessions could take the form of a series of training vignettes where the trainee is confronted with varying therapeutic encounters where standardized patients (such as those used in medical training scenarios) present transference-tinged information about the trainee. These sessions could even be done in a virtual reality format. The trainee could then observe and record his or her countertransference reactions while practicing how to process and/or use these reactions.

CHAPTER 4

Neutrality, transference, countertransference, counterresponse

Transference

Transference, generally speaking, is a naturally occurring displacement or projection of a pattern of relationship (this includes attitudes, feelings, thoughts, etc.) originally experienced in early childhood relationships. These early relationships with significant persons (usually caregivers or parental figures from early childhood, termed objects in psychoanalysis) are reexperienced throughout the person's adult life. Transference colors almost all human relationships to some degree, but transference-heavy relationships are almost always problematic or pathological. These transference-heavy relationships have been characterized as a *transference neurosis* (Greenson, 1967). This characterization is somewhat misleading because it implies the outdated belief that people with more severe mental illnesses such as personality disorders or psychosis do not form transference relationships. We now know this is not true (K. Volkan & V. D. Volkan, 2022; V. D. Volkan, 1987). Transference relationships are repetitive and unconscious, meaning that they occur without a person becoming aware of their repetitive nature. In psychoanalytic work, the patient's personality organization (which we will discuss later) plays an important role in the type of transference that manifests in psychotherapy. Patients can develop a transference neurosis, an intensive borderline transference, or a narcissistic transference. The resolution of these transferences leads to positive structural changes within the patient's mind.

In psychotherapy, transference relationships always occur with the therapist. This is true regardless of whether the type of psychotherapy addresses transference or not. In psychoanalysis and psychoanalytic psychotherapy, transference is used to understand the patterns that the patient brings into his or her relationships with others. Patients are not aware at a conscious level that transference is taking place. This means they are expressing feelings that are inaccessible to the conscious mind. The psychoanalytic clinician serves as a sort of movie screen that the patient unconsciously projects his or her transferential pattern of relationship onto. The psychoanalytic clinician can then decipher the pattern of the transference to give insights about the nature of the patient's problems. This will include the developmental level where the problems originated as well as patterns of relating that are typical for that developmental level. The psychoanalytic clinician will then interpret his or her insights to the patient. Over time, the patient will come to understand and be aware of his or her transference and how this affects his or her thoughts, behavior, and feelings. In other words, the process of psychoanalysis or psychoanalytic psychotherapy allows patients the opportunity to reexperience their important early relationships in a more satisfactory manner. Over time, as the psychoanalytic clinician interprets the transference patterns that the patient exhibits, the patient becomes more and more conscious of them. Eventually the patient begins to understand how his or her unconscious patterns of relating manifest outside the therapy hour. This starts to change how the patient interacts with others in general, leading to more satisfying connections to others and a greater capacity for intimacy.

Relationship as the cure

By maintaining neutrality, the psychoanalytic clinician does not react to the transference pattern in the same way as significant people in the patient's past. This requires the psychoanalytic clinician to become a consistent presence and slowly emerge as a new "analytic" object for the patient. This is accomplished through repeated and timely interpretation of the transference.

The psychoanalytic clinician, as a new analytic object, can foster more normalized psychological development (Akhtar, 2000). Over time the patient can internalize this more mature way of relating to others. This idea was first articulated as a corrective emotional experience by Franz Alexander and Thomas French (1946) in their early book on psychoanalytic psychotherapy. While the concept of psychotherapy as a corrective emotional experience has fallen out of favor in some psychoanalytic circles, it may play an important role in psychoanalytic psychotherapy, which is typically of shorter duration and depth than psychoanalysis.

Even though psychoanalytic psychotherapy may not result in personality change in the patient, it may be able to modify the way in which a patient interacts with others in a significant enough way to alleviate symptoms and allow him or her to live a more fulfilling life. There is now research demonstrating that psychotherapy does function as a corrective emotional experience, modifying the ways in which patients relate to others. Interestingly, a number of non-psychoanalytic as well as psychoanalytically derived psychotherapies have incorporated this idea even though they do not explicitly acknowledge the therapeutic role of working with transference (Gülüm & Soygüt, 2021; Nakamura et al., 2022; Peck, 2021).

Positive and negative transference

There are generally two kinds of transference—positive and negative. In positive transference, the patient projects his or her idealization of early objects onto the therapist. Often intense, the patient can over-idealize the therapist and/or develop strong feelings of love or sexual attraction toward the therapist. Positive transference typically manifests early in the therapeutic relationship.

Negative transference generally appears later. In negative transference, the patient can become critical, resentful, angry, hostile, or aggressive toward the therapist. While positive transference tends to arise first and negative transference later, there is a good deal of ambivalence in the transference. In other words, the transference can alternate between being positive and negative, depending on the pattern of relationship that is playing out in the therapy process. However, in the case of more severe mental illness, such as personality disorders that utilize splitting defenses, the contrast between positive and negative transference can be more absolute.

Case example of transference 1

A woman entered into psychoanalytic psychotherapy with a male therapist because she had troubles at work. She had a difficult time relating to her coworkers, who thought her somewhat aloof. However, she constantly sought out her male supervisor's attention to the point that he would avoid her if possible. When this woman couldn't get her supervisor's attention, she would end up getting sick and not come to work. Every time she called in sick, she was required to report it to her supervisor, who had to keep track of absences and admonish her to get a doctor's note. This woman had grown up as a middle child in a large family with several brothers and sisters. During her therapy sessions she revealed that her father worked long hours when she was a child, and she didn't see him very much. However, if she became ill, her father would put his work aside and take care of her, paying attention to her and not her siblings. During individual therapy sessions the woman would become somewhat cloying and annoying in her behavior, causing her therapist to dread sessions with the woman. The woman also participated in group therapy sessions with her male therapist and a female co-therapist. During group therapy, if she felt that the other group members received too much attention, she would often call in sick for subsequent sessions and request that the male therapist call her at home.

This case was interesting because it demonstrates how early relationships can be recreated by the patient. In this case, the woman used projective identification—that is, projecting qualities onto the therapist that made him behave and feel the way her rejecting father had done. In the group psychotherapy setting, when her fellow group members received attention from the male therapist, she would seek to get his attention in the same way she got her father's attention as a child. In this case, the male therapist was able to examine his countertransference reactions to understand the patient's transference neurosis. Over time, he was able to interpret the transference to the woman so she could understand that she was replaying out her early relationship with her father as well as resisting the psychotherapy process. The woman began to get along better at work and have a more realistic relationship with her boss. She was also able to start and develop genuine friendships with other group therapy members.

Centrality of the concept of transference

Regardless of the proliferation of many different types of psychother-apy over the years, it remains accurate to say that psychoanalysis and psychoanalytic psychotherapy, broadly defined, are the only types of psychotherapy that specifically work with transference. In other words, these are the only kinds of psychotherapy that examine the way in which patients recreate early childhood relationships that are maladaptive in adulthood, analyzing them to make the patient conscious of these rela-tionships, and then resolving these through repeated and timely inter-pretation as well as through a corrective (i.e., stable and consistent) relationship with the psychoanalytic clinician. It is also accurate to say that psychoanalysis proper, as opposed to psychoanalytic psychother-apy, is more likely to result in a relatively more systematic and complete resolution of transference reactions than psychoanalytic psychotherapy, which is much more variable in techniques used, treatment duration, and treatment intensity. Nevertheless, working with transference is still a key aspect of any psychoanalytic or psychoanalytic-adjacent psycho-therapy. As Freud stated in his work *On the History of the Psycho-Analytic Movement* (1914d),

> It may thus be said that the theory of psycho-analysis is an attempt to account for two striking and unexpected facts of observation which emerge whenever an attempt is made to trace the symptoms of a neurotic back to their sources in his past life: the facts of transference and of resistance. Any line of investigation which recognizes these two facts and takes them as the starting point of its work has a right to call itself psycho-analysis, even though it arrives at results other than my own. (p. 16)

The techniques of psychoanalysis and psychoanalytic psychotherapy work to encourage a transference regression whereby the patient reexperiences his or her early relationship patterns with the analyst or psychotherapist during the therapy session. Whatever can be said of non-psychoanalytic psychotherapies (and there are many good things that can be said), they do not work with transference, and hence do not permanently help patients stop the use of maladaptive childhood patterns of relating as an adult. Instead, many non-analytic therapies give patients the ability to repress transference reactions or even modify their life situations so that their transference reactions do not cause as much disruption in their lives, but they do not help resolve transference.

Case example of transference 2

A family therapist of our acquaintance was asked to see the daughter of a prominent couple. The father was a highly successful film industry executive, and the mother was a socialite. The father traveled quite a bit and did not spend much time at home. When he was home, he said he was usually too exhausted to give his children much attention. The mother was very involved in social activities and in keeping up the appearance of wealth. Her interactions with her children were mostly to get them to present the right image to her friends. The daughter, who was the oldest child, began to act out by using drugs and rebelling. After taking her father's Ferrari (without his permission) on a joyride and crashing it, she was given a choice of going to therapy or being required to attend a stricter school while living at home. The therapist quite appropriately required the parents to accompany their daughter to group therapy sessions, in addition to the individual therapy the daughter received. The therapist quickly realized that the parents were the ones with serious psychological issues and that the daughter's acting out was actually a rational attempt to get help. Over the course of a year, the therapist became a consistent parental object for the girl, encouraging her to go to college and become independent of her parents (who had dropped out of therapy after only a few sessions). The girl was able to go away to college in a distant city and subsequently live on her own. While she was able to graduate from the university and get a job, she reportedly had difficulties in her relationships with her professors and work supervisors.

This case is a good example of how a non-analytic therapist helped a patient repress her transference reactions and adapt her life situation so that transference reactions caused minimal disruption to her life. However, it is highly likely that as an adult, this patient will use the same patterns she developed as a child to survive in her relationship with her inadequate parents. This will likely be maladaptive, and she will eventually require more psychotherapy.

Transference takes on specific patterns related to unresolved developmental conflicts. These patterns are associated with the developmental stage where the pattern originates and are shaped by the patient's level of personality organization. For instance, a common pattern of transference is associated with the Oedipus complex. This complex, which we will describe below, is triadic in the sense that it originated in the patient's relationship with his or her father and mother. In more severe mental states, the transference patterns may be more dyadic, originating through the relationship of the patient with his or her primary mothering figure in infancy. Dyadic transference patterns are more difficult to bring to conscious awareness because they originate when the patient was at a preverbal level, and the transference patterns consist more of feelings than thoughts. Our discussion of transference highlights the importance of understanding the development level and personality organization of the patient, discussed further on.

Neutrality

As discussed previously, therapeutic identity, besides paying attention to confidentiality, depends on the concept of *neutrality*. In 1915 Freud mentioned "neutrality" while referring to a psychoanalyst's attitude toward his or her patients. As Alex Hoffer (1985) and Ernest Wallwork (2005) remind us, the German word Freud used for this concept was "*Indifferenz*," rather than "*Neutralitaet*," the German word for "neutrality." While translating Freud's works into English (*The Standard Edition of the Complete Psychological Works of Sigmund*

Freud, Vol. 1–24), James Strachey used the English word "neutrality," thereafter replacing "indifference" as the term accepted in the English psychoanalytic literature.

Sigmund Freud's clear description of this concept can be found in his 1919 paper, "Lines of Advances in Psychoanalytic Therapy," in which he refers to avoiding turning a patient "into our private property, to decide his fate for him, to force our own ideals on him, and with the pride of a Creator to form him in our own image and to see that it is good" (p. 164).

Anna Freud (1936) described neutrality as meaning a stance equidistant from the demands of the id, ego, and superego. In later years, this description was criticized, especially by ego psychologists, who perceive psychoanalysts to be on the side of the patient's ego with the goal of helping patients enrich it. As one might expect, the meaning of therapeutic neutrality has been discussed throughout the decades by many analysts from different schools of psychoanalysis (see, for example: Adler & Bachant, 1996; Agatsuma, 2014; Bornstein, 1983; Gill, 1994; Glover, 1955; Greenson, 1958; Kernberg, 1976; Klautau & Coelho, 2013; Kris, 1982; Laplanche & Pontalis, 1973; Poland, 1984; Shapiro, 1984; Stone, 1961).

During the last few decades, the concept of neutrality has been linked with the concept of countertransference. Burness Moore and Bernard Fine (1990) wrote:

> Central to psychoanalytic neutrality are keeping the countertransference in check, avoiding the imposition of one's own values upon the patient, and taking the patient's capacities rather than one's own desires as a guide. … The psychoanalyst's neutrality is intended to facilitate the development, recognition, and interpretation of the transference neurosis and to minimize distortions that might be introduced if he or she attempts to educate, advise, or impose values upon the patient based on the psychoanalyst's countertransference. (p. 127)

Michael and Batya Shoshani (2021) remind us that the psychoanalytic stance of technical neutrality may be interpreted differently by different patients. For example, referring to Sándor Ferenczi's (2012) observations, they state that patients who had been traumatized may interpret the psychotherapist's therapeutic neutrality as rejection and desertion. When a psychotherapist senses this, it will be important for him or her to make appropriate remarks illustrating that his or her technical approach does not mean rejection or desertion.

Rachel Blass (2003) and Ernest Wallwork (2005) examined therapeutic neutrality from an ethical point of view. Nancy Hollander (2009) reminded us of "ethical non-neutrality" when psychoanalysts need to address psychological destructive processes that manifest in the world; she was not, however, speaking about non-neutrality in the clinical setting. Due to the importance of therapeutic neutrality, a practicing psychoanalytic clinician needs to be careful when making public remarks, such as in the media, about events that take place outside of a therapeutic office.

As previously discussed, the decreasing ability of psychotherapists to maintain privacy about their non-therapeutic lives due to the internet and social media impacts their ability to use therapeutic neutrality. Although some psychoanalytic clinicians who hail from relational and interpersonal schools have modified the idea of neutrality, even modifying the restriction of self-disclosure and self-revelation to some degree, this is still not meant to extinguish the therapists' sense of privacy about their own lives, nor to constrain the possibilities of what can be said in the therapeutic space because of private information from the therapist (Kaluzeviciute, 2020).

Neutrality has fallen out of favor in some psychoanalytic circles, especially among relational psychoanalysts and psychoanalytic psychotherapists. But this is due, in part at least, to a shallow understanding of neutrality. For many of these clinicians, neutrality is equated with a cold aloofness where the clinician is rather robotic and acts somewhat superior to his or her patients. This view of neutrality at least partly originates in Freud's analogy comparing psychoanalysis to surgery, in which the surgeon must put aside all his human feelings to operate (Freud, 1912). However, as Charles Gelso and Katri Kanninen (2017) point out,

> It is very easy to pull from these assertions that the analyst should be distant, aloof, and without feelings for the patient. However, as anyone who has studied Freud knows, these quotes were only part of the story, for Freud elsewhere underscored the importance of the analyst's caring, empathy, and engagement in a real relationship with the analysand. (p. 331)

Gelso and Kanninen go on to outline a therapeutic neutrality that is not aloof, indifferent, or passive. They identify five characteristics of effective neutrality. The first is that the therapist needs to function as an observer seeking to understand the patient and his or her relationship to the patient. This requires the therapist to function with dual attention to the patient and the relationship with the patient. The second characteristic entails not taking sides. In other words, the therapist tries to position themselves equidistant from the patient's id, ego, and superego. The therapist does not side with the patient's wishes and impulses, nor does he or she make moral judgments and determinations or side with the admonition or control of the patient's impulses and wishes. The third characteristic expands the second vis-à-vis the therapist not taking sides in the patient's outer struggles. The therapist's job is to help patients understand their feelings about the people and situations in their life, not to advocate like a lawyer for patients' particular positions. The fourth characteristic of neutrality involves the therapist modulating his or her own affects while refraining from manipulating the affects of his or her patients. This includes things like not exuding excessive warmth or manipulating the patient into a catharsis such as crying. The fifth and last characteristic requires the therapist to carry out therapy in a state of abstinence, that is, not responding to patients' demands for affection, dependency, requests, etc.

Abstinence

In psychoanalysis, "abstinence" is also examined as an aspect of "neutrality." In 1915, Freud wrote:

> The treatment must be carried out in abstinence. By this I do not mean physical abstinence alone, nor yet the deprivation of everything that the patient desires, for perhaps no sick patient could tolerate this. Instead, I shall state it as a fundamental principle that the patient's need and longing should be allowed to persist in her, in order that they may serve as forces impelling her to do work and make changes. (1915a, p. 165)

Some psychoanalytic clinicians, such as those who are followers of "relational psychoanalysis," found ambiguity in Freud's statement

(Poland, 1984; Schlesinger, 2003). "Relational psychoanalysis" began in the 1980s in the United States and put more emphasis on a child's relationship with the mothering person in developing the mind and generally disregarded the Freudian emphasis on instinctual drives (S. A. Mitchell, 1988, 2000). During treatment, relational psychoanalytic clinicians seem to ignore or pay less attention to the motivation for the patient's free associations, focusing instead on the patient's relationships. Relational psychoanalysts and psychotherapists no longer see the need for drives. Instead, they believe in a "drive" to be in relationships. For these clinicians, it is important to have an authentic presence when working with patients so they can experience the relationship. Because of this, Freud's classical ideas of neutrality are rejected, and the therapist is given leeway to disclose more about themselves with the idea that this will make the relationship with the therapist more "real." This leads relational clinicians to place less emphasis on free association and making interpretations, as well as on maintaining neutrality, anonymity, and abstinence (Schill, 2004).

In our opinion, abandoning the drives does a disservice to the patient. While relationships are important, understanding what motivates relationships tells us a lot about their nature and the nature of the transference that accompanies them. Many relational psychoanalytic clinicians seem to rely on concepts such as John Bowlby's attachment styles (1978), which, while important, certainly arise from underlying mental patterns fueled by pleasure-seeking, aggression/frustration, and the anxiety that arises from these feelings. These mental patterns contain representations of significant others that then become the basis for later relationships with actual people. Ignoring these mental patterns (which are called object relations) and how they are motivated by the drives will result in an incomplete understanding of the nature of the patient's relationships and how the patient's pattern of relating plays out with his or her psychoanalytic clinician. Allowing self-disclosure under the pretense of being more real only serves to contaminate the transference and to allow for more unexamined countertransference. We can also question whether more self-disclosure results in a more real, authentic relationship with the patient. As Michael Schill (2004) says,

> Analysis requires the patient to accept that people in everyday life are extremely unlikely to be as consistently empathic and

understanding as the analyst, or to be as able or interested in explaining their way of thinking and feeling to the patient as an analyst might. (p. 162)

In fact, a more authentic relationship with the patient may be realized with a psychoanalytic clinician who maintains neutrality and abstinence. This can help the patient understand that the analytic/therapeutic situation is not the same as "real life." A more self-disclosing therapist may cause the patient to mistake the therapeutic situation, which has a specific purpose, for a friendship or other non-analytic relationship.

Salman Akhtar (2009) summarizes the principle of abstinence by stating that psychoanalysts neither attempt to modify the transference by indulging the patient nor by focusing on their own view of who they actually are. But he also reminds us that abstinence can coexist when the psychoanalyst sometimes makes remarks to encourage and support the patient's analytic ego.

In the *Ethics Case Book of the American Psychoanalytic Association*, edited by Paul Dewald and Rita Clark (2001), there is a story of a female patient who experienced great sadness accompanied by uncontrollable sobbing during a session in the second year of her analysis. Her psychoanalyst put his arm around this patient's shoulder as she got up from the couch, held her briefly, and attempted to comfort her. In the next session, the patient made no reference to this experience. Dewald and Clark's book goes on to discuss how a psychoanalyst would handle unexpected boundary-crossing situations. The discussion concludes that if a patient does not bring up such an experience the psychoanalyst should inquire about the patient's response to it and explore with the patient what it meant to her.

Decades ago, Viviana, a beautiful woman who was having certain marital problems, became Vamık Volkan's analysand. She lived in another city but drove for over an hour to his office four times a week. She started her third session on the couch by asking her psychoanalyst to meet with her in a motel four times a week instead of the office and have a good time. Vamık Volkan responded by telling her that if he agreed to do what she was asking she would face a great loss. This response puzzled her. She demanded to know what her loss would be. He said, "You will lose me as your psychoanalyst." After this interaction, Viviana was able to start developing a therapeutic alliance.

Abstinence also includes not drinking, eating, or—contrary to Freud's practice—smoking during the sessions.

Patient abstinence

In addition to the abstinence practised by the psychotherapist, it is important for patients to maintain some abstinence. The usual admonition in psychoanalysis and for many other types of psychotherapy is that patients resist making impulsive impactful life changes while undergoing therapy. It is to be made clear that it is important not to initiate a move, a divorce, or even a major purchase of stocks, etc., while in therapy until psychological factors related to such decisions are understood and assimilated. Writing at a time when most psychoanalytic clinicians were psychiatrists, Frieda Fromm-Reichmann (1950) states,

> The decision for engagement, marriage, or divorce or any such crucial steps in a patient's life should be discouraged by the psychiatrist while the patient is under intensive psychotherapy. The goal of psychotherapy is a change in the patient's personality. Neither he or the psychiatrist can know ahead of time what the result of this change will be. It is to be assumed, therefore, that the patient is in no position to know whether commitments made prior to this change may prove desirable in the future. In some cases it is so obvious that the psychiatrist is justified in demanding outright that such decisions be postponed. He may even go so far, at times, as to deem it advisable that treatment be discontinued if the patient does not follow his suggestion. The postponement of all vital decisions until treatment has been terminated is one of the basic rules in classical psychoanalysis. (p. 204)

However, there may be situations where the patient is already in the midst of a process or in the middle of making a life decision when they enter therapy. For instance, a patient might be engaged with a wedding date set and venue paid for, or a patient might already be pregnant. In fact, the import of a decision can be the reason the patient enters therapy in the first place. In these cases, the psychoanalytic clinician will need to weigh the injunction of patient abstinence with the potential for impeding progress in the patient's life. It will be important in such cases for the psychoanalytic clinician and the patient to explore and clarify any unconscious motivations behind any life-changing decisions. The astute psychoanalytic clinician should also investigate whether any breach of patient abstinence is a form of unconscious acting out on the part of the patient that is often a manifestation of transference.

There are also major events that occur that are out of the patient's control. Fromm-Reichmann (1950) also wrote about the impact of major events in the patient's life and how these should be dealt with. These events include occurrences that the patient has control over and some that he or she does not. Examples include pregnancy, childbirth, marriage, divorce, the death of a close relative, severe illness, accidents, natural disasters, war, as well as suicidal attempts. In general, she allows that the psychoanalytic clinician may break from his or her therapeutic stance and offer words of condolences, concern, or in the case of pregnancy, congratulations.

In any event, it is incumbent on the psychoanalytic clinician to acknowledge that the occurrence, whatever it may be, is a significant event in the patient's life. It is also important for the psychoanalytic clinician to have some understanding of how the patient feels in light of the occurrence of a major event. Not all patients will experience the death of a relative as negative or the advent of pregnancy as positive. The psychoanalytic clinician needs to be very sensitive to this.

Fromm-Reichmann writes a good deal regarding the pregnancy of the patient. She does not see the continuation of therapy during pregnancy as a negative.

> In my opinion it is preferable, *as a rule*, to clarify potentially disturbing emotional factors in the life of a pregnant woman rather than to leave this material undiscussed and free to influence a patient one way or another outside her knowledge and, therefore, outside her control. Clarification may be for the benefit of the expectant mother as well as for the benefit of the child which she carries. (p. 203)

According to Fromm-Reichmann, these potentially disturbing factors are often related to the pregnant woman's relationship to her own mother. Clarifying these factors can be of great importance during and after the pregnancy.

Counterresponse

While supervising psychoanalytic clinicians, on many occasions we hear these clinicians refer to every thought or action related to their patients as their countertransference. We have already discussed the classical description of countertransference above. As Karl Menninger wrote long ago, it refers to the inability "to understand certain kinds of material which touch upon the psychoanalyst's own personal problems" (Menninger, 1958, p. 88).

We previously discussed the case from Paul Dewald and Rita Clark's (2001) edited book in which a male psychoanalyst touched his female patient. The role of the psychoanalyst's countertransference in such a boundary-crossing is clear. We are informed that the psychoanalyst was recalling some of his own troubled childhood experiences while his patient was talking and sobbing, and this led him to touch his patient and try to comfort her with bodily contact.

There are occasions when a psychoanalytic clinician makes remarks that interfere with his or her therapeutic neutrality and abstinence that are not related to the clinician's countertransference. Instead, they represent "counterresponses" to events that must be corrected to protect the therapeutic process. We separate the term countertransference from the term counterresponse. In the psychoanalytic literature, there are huge numbers of papers on countertransference, but "counterresponse" has not been referred to often. The following case illustrates counterresponse and how it can be addressed in psychotherapy.

Case example of counterresponse

Charles, a young man, felt that he was falling in love with the secretary of his boss, a woman of his age. He also had a fantasy that his boss was having a sexual affair with the secretary. This caused Charles to stay away from the young woman, and he felt angry and depressed. This affected his work performance, and he lost his job. Because of this, Charles started psychotherapy. His psychotherapist noted that this young man had oedipal issues stemming from his childhood.

When Charles had been in therapy for about six months, the psychotherapist's wife told her husband that often she would see a car parked in front of their house with a young man sitting in it. When she went shopping, she would see the same young man following her. She gave a description of this young man. The psychotherapist wondered if Charles was the person who was following his wife. The patient had not mentioned such an activity. When the psychotherapist asked Charles if he was the one following his wife, he quickly admitted that he was the follower. Hearing this, the psychotherapist said to his patient: "Our therapeutic relationship is between you and me. You will stop following my wife right away. If you do not stop, I will no longer be your psychotherapist and I will call the police." Charles stopped following the psychotherapist's wife and his treatment continued.

Sometimes it is difficult to separate counterresponse from countertransference. However, counterresponse primarily is a response to real world issues that the patient or the therapist faces whether they induce aspects of the therapist's childhood experiences and responses or not. A good example of this is when a female psychotherapist becomes pregnant.

According to Fromm-Reichmann (1950), if a significant occurrence takes place in the life of the therapist, treatment should be continued as long as the therapist does not feel that whatever is going on will affect his or her ability to conduct psychotherapy. If the patient notices that something is different or off, the therapist can make a simple direct statement of the facts, then saying that whatever is going on will not affect their work together. On the other hand, the patient may feel that whatever is going on with the therapist is a significant disruption or it may be that whatever is going on is so disruptive that the therapist feels that he or she cannot effectively render therapy. In this case,

> It may be advisable for the psychiatrist to interrupt treatment for a sufficiently long period of time to take care of his preoccupation with his own affairs. As treatment is resumed, he may unassumingly comment upon his reasons for the interruption and add that he is ready for work. (Fromm-Reichmann, 1950, p. 210)

CHAPTER 5

The psychoanalytic clinician's office

A psychoanalytic clinician's office and everything within it is a psychological extension of the therapist. It should be designed in a way that helps the psychoanalytic clinician hold on to his or her therapeutic identity as well as therapeutic neutrality, confidentiality, and abstinence. It should be easily accessible, stable, and comfortable.

Couch vs. chair

The use of the couch has become a key signifier of psychoanalysis. For some, having the patient recline on the couch during the session is what determines whether psychoanalysis or some sort of psychoanalytic psychotherapy is being done. However, the reality is more complicated. The ostensible aim of a psychoanalyst's sitting behind his or her couch and the patient not seeing him or her helps the patient to speak freely and develop workable transferences. The couch also allows the patient to relax, which, in turn, fosters a more or less hypnogogic state that more easily enables unconscious content to surface.

For the psychoanalyst, using the couch is a central technique. It can also be a source of pride and a way of anchoring a professional identity.

Psychoanalysts undergo their training analysis on the couch. Its use is baked into their character. Use of the couch can also be a fixed point for the psychoanalyst who must contend with what is essentially the improvisatory process of psychoanalysis. In fact, use of the couch may be so ingrained that it is often used by psychoanalysts to conduct psychoanalytic psychotherapy.

Kevin Volkan underwent psychoanalytic psychotherapy as part of his training. His psychoanalytic psychotherapy was conducted by a psychoanalyst with his sessions on the couch while she sat behind him, as is standard psychoanalytic practice. The only difference between her approach and psychoanalysis proper was the frequency of visits. We have also heard and observed psychoanalysts from various schools who do not use the couch but conduct analysis face-to-face.

On the other hand, in our experience, it is very rare to find psychoanalytic psychotherapists that use the couch. We are sure they are out there, but we have not come across them. For psychoanalytic psychotherapists, use of the couch is not part of their identity and is rarely part of their training. Even if a psychoanalytic psychotherapist wanted to use the couch, there is a fear that this would be professionally frowned upon since the common understanding is that the couch is the province only of fully trained psychoanalysts. However, there is no absolute restriction preventing psychoanalytic psychotherapists from using the couch.

When Kevin Volkan, who is not an analyst, saw patients, he did not use the couch. Instead, he would vary where his patients were placed depending on their level of pathology. For higher-functioning patients, he used chairs but did not have them face the therapist. He would angle the patient's chair away, so they were not looking directly at the therapist. Patients with more severe psychopathology would have their chair angled to face the therapist more directly. Angling the chairs greatly facilitated free association and provided a couch-like experience that could be adjusted for more severely disturbed patients to provide more structure. This deviation of technique derives from the British psychoanalyst Ronald Fairbairn, who thought of the couch as a holdover from Freud's dislike of being looked at and his initial forays into hypnosis (Fairbairn, 1958). He sought to come up with a sitting arrangement that would facilitate free association and yet encourage an optimal therapeutic alliance. As Fairbairn said,

> … I do not favour the technique of the face-to-face interview … In actual practice I sit at a desk, and the patient sits in a comfortable chair placed to the side of the desk, almost parallel to mine, but slightly inclined towards me. In terms of this arrangement, patient and analyst are not ordinarily looking at one another; but either may look at the other if he so wishes. Thus the setting of an object-relationship is maintained without undue embarrassment to either party … my personal experience is that the demands of the patient are actually less exacting when he is not isolated from the analyst on the couch and thus deprived of any real relationship with him. (p. 378)

For patients with more severe issues, such as borderline personality disorders or even psychoses, psychoanalysts will generally use the couch. However, this isn't always true. Some psychoanalysts will forgo using the couch with patients suffering from more severe mental problems. The psychoanalyst Otto Kernberg, for instance, often worked face-to-face with patients suffering from borderline personality disorder. This was done in order to facilitate more of a therapeutic container (Kernberg, 1975, 1984a). The use of face-to-face psychotherapy as a therapeutic container was especially important for one of Kevin Volkan's patients who suffered from borderline personality disorder and would become psychotic anytime she became challenged or stressed in therapy.

Psychoanalytic psychotherapists who see their patients face-to-face may put a table between the comfortable chairs where they and their patients sit and put a box of tissues on the table. Some patients may need tissues if they cry.

Personal items

We suggest that psychoanalytic clinicians should not hang their family pictures in their offices. This protects confidentiality and avoids interfering with the patients' developing fantasies about their psychotherapists and their families related to transference expectations.

In the book *Psychoanalytic Technique Expanded: A Textbook on Psychoanalytic Treatment* (V. D. Volkan, 2010), Vamık Volkan wrote about a young psychoanalyst who hung an antique sword on the wall next to his couch. In Volkan's role as clinical supervisor, he did not know of the existence of this sword. Later, when he learned about the sword, he realized how the young analyst's male patient with castration anxiety was having difficulty working through his problems while lying on the couch and looking at the sword above him.

Many patients show attention to potted plants in their psychotherapists' offices. For example, while recalling deprivation of motherly love, they become preoccupied with how their psychotherapists take care of the plants.

Case example of personal items

During her first session with a psychotherapist, Natalie spoke of her traumatic childhood experiences. The psychotherapist noted how this patient was dealing with the lack of motherly love during childhood. Because of this, she was struggling to develop a stable, but narcissistic, sense of self. Natalie described how she surrounded herself with the "best" paintings, "fantastic" dinner plates, or sweets at her home. During the first session with this patient, the psychotherapist noted her counter-response; she thought that this new patient would regard her office as not good enough. In fact, Natalie focused on one area of the carpet in the psychotherapist's office and named it a "black spot."

Two weeks later, during the supervision session, the psychotherapist easily understood how her patient had externalized her love-hungry childhood self-image on this "black spot." However, it turned out that the psychotherapist had already removed the carpet from her office since her patient had found it "dirty" or "bad." It is important to keep the items in the office stable since any big change in the furniture may interfere with the developing transference expectations or, if the psychotherapy had been going for some time, with the existing transference stories.

Remote sessions

A major external factor, the spread of Covid-19 and its variants, has made it necessary for psychoanalysts and psychotherapists to conduct treatment while their patients are not present in their offices. The International Psychoanalytical Association and other psychoanalytic associations provided guidelines for distance treatment by taking advantage of phone or online technologies. Some psychoanalysts have already written about the impact of this drastic change to psychoanalytic treatment (Blackman, 2020; Lombardi, 2020; Prince, 2021; V. D. Volkan, 2021c). Our suggestion for psychoanalytic clinicians is to keep regular accepted hours for online treatment and clarify, and when it is appropriate, interpret, the patient's individualized responses to not being in the psychoanalyst's or psychotherapist's office. We note that stopping in-person sessions has played a role in increasing communications outside the set therapy hours, such as patients' leaving many text messages for their clinician. We suggest that psychoanalytic clinicians therapeutically handle this situation and keep communications within the agreed upon therapy hours. It is too early to know how this new experience, along with incredibly rapid developments in communication technology, will impact how psychoanalysis and psychoanalytic psychotherapy will be conducted after the virus pandemic is over. Nevertheless, we are seeing grief reactions in patients who were suddenly deprived of face-to-face therapy hours, as well as defensive reactions related to the dangerousness and anxiety created by Covid-19.

CHAPTER 6

Developmental levels

All the world's a stage,
And all the men and women merely players;
They have their exits and their entrances,
And one man in his time plays many parts,
His acts being seven ages. At first the infant,
Mewling and puking in the nurse's arms.
Then, the whining school-boy with his satchel
And shining morning face, creeping like snail
Unwillingly to school. And then the lover,
Sighing like furnace, with a woeful ballad
Made to his mistress' eyebrow. Then, a soldier,
Full of strange oaths, and bearded like the pard,
Jealous in honour, sudden, and quick in quarrel,
Seeking the bubble reputation
Even in the cannon's mouth. And then, the justice,
In fair round belly, with a good capon lined,
With eyes severe, and beard of formal cut,
Full of wise saws, and modern instances,
And so he plays his part. The sixth age shifts
Into the lean and slippered pantaloon,
With spectacles on nose and pouch on side,
His youthful hose, well saved, a world too wide

For his shrunk shank, and his big manly voice,
Turning again toward childish treble, pipes
And whistles in his sound. Last scene of all,
That ends this strange eventful history,
Is second childishness and mere oblivion,
Sans teeth, sans eyes, sans taste, sans everything.
—*As You Like It*, Act 2, Scene 7, lines 140–167
(Shakespeare, 1623)

The stages of human life have been contemplated throughout history. As the above quote from Shakespeare indicates, there are distinct stages or levels that we go through in our lifetimes. These levels have unique characteristics that define our existence. However, it wasn't until Sigmund Freud that the mechanisms by which one level evolved to the next were explained.

Sigmund Freud (1905d, 1923e, 1933a) described the psychosexual development of an individual. Freud explained the human journey through the different developmental levels via an understanding of sexual drive theory and the erogenous areas of the body. Today, psychoanalytic clinicians refer to five steps of the Freudian psychosexual ladder: the oral, the anal, the phallic, the latent, and the genital. Freud himself only mentioned four steps and did not name the latency period. Let us start examining the development of the human mind by looking at the Freudian ladder.

Freudian developmental levels

Oral phase

The oral phase starts at birth and lasts throughout the first eighteen months of life. Karl Abraham (1924) subdivided this phase into two periods: oral-erotic and oral-aggressive. During the oral-erotic period, while the infant sucks the breast, his or her sexual and aggressive drives are not yet differentiated. During the oral-aggressive period, the baby sometimes bites the breast, illustrating the separation of sexual and aggressive drives. He or she starts sensing what is ambivalence.

Freud described how fixation to the oral phase can take place when the infant's oral needs are not satisfied or are met excessively. He connected an adult's nail biting, smoking, excessive drinking, and chewing gum to such a fixation. Later psychoanalytic clinicians linked other psychological conditions during adulthood such as addiction, depression, extreme dependency or extreme generosity, and extreme optimism to oral phase fixations. Karl Menninger (1958) described how "oral erotization" of the analysis becomes observable.

> For some patients every word of the analyst is a pearl; for others, their own words are spoken as if they are minting gold coins with their lips. Pleasure from aggressive oral tendencies is sometimes clearly, although unpleasantly, detectable in the spitting or biting nature of the content or delivery of the patient's material. (p. 115)

Anal phase

The anal phase refers to the time period from twelve months to between eighteen and thirty-six months of life, during which a baby deals with issues linked to defecating or keeping feces inside and starts having a sense of independence. An adult's retentiveness or excessive generosity, stubbornness, unrestrained ambivalence, and obsessional behavior are expressions of this anal period of life.

In the clinical setting, we notice anal issues when a patient may act as if to say, "I will not move my bowels for you—unless ..." or "See, I move my bowels for you," or "I would if only you could ... please help me," or "Help me get started," or "Please give me an enema" (Menninger, 1958, p. 115).

An obsessional male patient of Vamık Volkan's provides a good example of issues stemming from this developmental phase. This patient would stay rather silent and talk about this or that event he had heard or read about in a newspaper without any emotion. He would be like a child experiencing constipation. Five or ten minutes prior to the ending of his sessions, his verbal and emotional constipation would disappear, and he would start telling the therapist with excitement about his dreams. Then, with a smile on his face, he would leave my office. This would make Volkan feel as if he was drenched with his diarrhea.

Phallic phase and oedipal issues

During the third phase of Freudian psychosexual development, between three to six years of age, children learn and focus on differences between male and female bodies. In male children, instinctual drives are invested into the penis; in female children, they are linked to the clitoris and vulva. During this phase, children dress and undress and explore the genital areas.

During the latter part of the phallic phase, the Oedipus complex, erotic interest in the opposite-sex parent and sexual rivalry with the same-sex parent appear and then are resolved. Freud (1905d, 1925j) described castration anxiety in male children and penis envy in female children during this phase.

During this developmental period, boys start having an unconscious sexual desire for their mothers. They are unconsciously motivated to see their fathers as rivals and want to get rid of them. However, they begin to fear that their father knows this and will castrate them. During normal development, boys are able to repress their feelings and then identify with the father. Later in life, most boys will go on to find a satisfactory female partner. It should be noted that most psychoanalytic clinicians do not ascribe pathology to gay people regarding the resolution of the oedipal phase. One idea is that boys who have a predisposition to homosexuality because of their biology may view their father as a primary erotic target and identify with their mothers. For a nuanced and long-overdue discussion of this subject, see Arthur Fox's paper "Gay-friendly Psychoanalysis and the Abiding Pleasures of Prejudice" (2018).

The pattern is a bit different for girls. Little girls are also in love with their mothers. But a little girl will notice her own lack of a penis, which gives rise to wanting to obtain one, that is, she develops what Freud termed "penis envy." However, once she realizes the impossibility of obtaining a penis, she transfers her desire to obtaining a baby as a substitute.

Freud thought that a girl resents her mother for not giving her a penis. He also suggested that since girls do not fear castration, they develop weaker superegos. Later psychoanalytic thinking has modified Freud's views by realizing that Freud did consider that boys' and girls' investments in their genital areas are different.

Penis envy

The central concept of the oedipal cycle for girls is the idea of penis envy. This has proven to be quite controversial. As most psychoanalytic clinicians will tell you, the phenomenon that has been labeled "penis envy" is extremely common, even if the standard Freudian interpretation of the phenomenon is not. In fact, there have been several different interpretations of the penis envy phenomenon. For instance, feminist psychoanalysts interpret penis envy as the little girl's growing awareness that she is denied the power and privilege given to males. Another interpretation is that the little girl envies the power of the mother to have the father's penis inside her. The girl then wants to possess a penis in order to satisfy the mother (Zepf, 2015).

The psychoanalyst Karen Horney, in her paper titled "On the Genesis of the Castration Complex in Women," which she presented in 1922 at the International Psychoanalytic Congress in Berlin and later published as a chapter in her book *Feminine Psychology* (1967), delves into three causes of penis envy in girls. The first is envy over what is termed *urethral eroticism*. This is the enjoyment boys get from producing a stream of urine, to which are attached omnipotent and sadistic fantasies. (This is reminiscent of little boys behaving like a god of destruction while urinating on an anthill.) The second cause of envy is exhibitionism on the part of the little boy, who gets to display his genitals and even admire them himself. For Horney, this jealousy of male exhibitionism is the root cause of later female display involving the whole body, including revealing clothing, jewelry, makeup, etc. The third cause for penis envy is that boys get to hold their genitals while urinating, which little girls construe as permission to masturbate. The little girl gets admonished for touching herself while the little boy has no such restriction.

While elaborating on penis envy in ways Freud did not necessarily approve of, Horney reaffirms the phenomenon of penis envy without considering women to be lesser than males. She can see and work with the phenomenon clinically without having to place women in a subordinate, less-than role. In other words, women are more than just men who do not possess penises. Horney promotes a sort of equality of jealousy between the sexes with both boys and girls having fantasies and desires for parental love and mutual envy for each other.

In a later paper titled *The Dread of Women,* originally published in 1932 in the *International Journal of Psychoanalysis* and also included as a chapter in *Feminine Psychology* (1967), Horney introduced the concept of womb envy as a counterpart to penis envy. While Horney did not coin the term womb envy, other writers applied the term to her ideas (Kittay, 1984; Mead, 1949). Basically, womb envy occurs when a boy realizes that he does not possess the creative power of his mother. In other words, he can never have a baby. Freud himself alluded to the male desire to bear children or to have female genitals—in his case, subjects Little Hans, Judge Schreber, and the Wolf Man (Freud, 1909b, 1911c, 1918b).

Children are aware of, and create unconscious fantasies around, their mother's pregnancies. The child's fantasies about the mother's pregnancy is related to their unborn siblings and the possibility of losing their mother's love (V. D. Volkan & Ast, 1997). For the male child, however, the pregnant mother also brings awareness that he doesn't possess the creative power of the mother. This leads to envy and anger. As he grows older, this takes the form of devaluing the feminine and evolves into misogyny. As female psychoanalysts have pointed out, psychoanalysis has tremendous explanatory power for understanding why women, in particular, have been devalued (Chodorow, 1978a, 1978b; Kittay, 1984; J. Mitchell, 1974).

In addition to the concept of womb envy, Nancy Chodorow has introduced the concept of the reproduction of mothering that gives more detail to girls' identification with the role of mothering (Chodorow, 1978a). As she puts it, "Women mother daughters who, when they become women, mother" (p. 209). Little girls identify with women who are their mothers, while their sons do not develop the same capacity for nurture because this capacity is inhibited or repressed. Womb envy is one possible explanation for this, while evolutionary fitness is another. Interestingly, noted primatologist Frans de Waal has commented on imitation in chimpanzees that resembles the reproduction of mothering in humans:

> … imitation is very interesting from the perspective of the gender studies that I'm involved in at the moment, in that I think there is a tendency for males to imitate males more, and for females to

imitate females more ... For example, young daughters, they copy the behavior of their moms more faithfully than young sons, and so there is this picking up of the model of your own sex, so to speak. (Carroll, 2022, 11:08)

We have included a lengthy discussion on the more nuanced view of penis envy because the oedipal stage of development is extremely important in conducting psychotherapy. Also, we believe it is worthwhile to attempt to redress the male-centric interpretation of this developmental stage that is common in Freudian psychology. We also recognize that most psychoanalytic clinicians these days are female. It is highly likely that if you are reading this book, you are a woman. In the last fifty years, the psychoanalytic and psychotherapy profession has gone from being made up mostly of men to being female-dominated (C.-H. Lin et al., 2008; Ludwig-Körner, 2021; Olos & Hoff, 2006). Therefore, understanding oedipal patterns from a female perspective is imperative to the profession.

The superego
Before children climb up to the next step of the psychological ladder, they identify with their parental figures. This results in their developing their superegos and ego ideals. We can imagine the concept of ego ideal as a counterpart of the superego. Salman Akhtar (2009) writes:

> The ego-ideal exhorts and pushes, striving to diminish the gap between the self as it is and as it desired to be. The superego, in contrast, criticizes one for transgressing inner moral injunctions. Failure to meet superego demands causes guilt. Failure to approach the ego-ideal's demands causes dejection and shame. (p. 89)

In the clinical setting, we notice the phallic step of the Freudian developmental stages when our patients become interested in the clinician's genital organ and desire to own it. For instance, there was a male patient who would walk into the office as if his body was an erect penis. There was also a female patient who spent many hours fantasizing about marrying the therapist and imagining the size of his penis. If the clinician is female, the patient may be preoccupied with the clinician's ability to bear children or capture a penis. This can engender rage in the patient if she suffers from the inability to do these things. Arrogance, exaggerated self-confidence, or an opposite psychic state such as easily injured vanity are linked to this phallic (or perhaps we should term it more generally as the genital) phase. Oedipal pathology may cause a man's preoccupation with competition with another man, usually an older one. It can also play out in sibling rivalries (V. D. Volkan & Ast, 1997). In adulthood, extreme jealousy, fear of authority figures, fear of intimacy, anxiety while having intercourse, searching for unsuitable partners such as a much older person, and some sexual deviations are also connected with oedipal issues. Later in this book, some case histories will illustrate how we observe phallic and oedipal issues in the clinical setting.

Before describing the next step of the developmental ladder, the latency phase, we wish to state that the superego concept is not an easy one to apply to a clinical situation unless the patient in analysis has a cohesive self-representation and his or her conflicts are primarily centered upon oedipal problems. In other words, the patient has a neurotic personality organization (we will describe different personality organizations later in this book). To deal with the difficulty of using the term "superego" in relation to patients—including those with a neurotic personality organization whose superegos have not been fully integrated to one degree or another—psychoanalysts use many different adjectives to be more specific about what kind of superego they are referring to. Thus, in the psychoanalytic literature we reference "forerunners of the superego," "precursors of the superego," "archaic superego," "regression in some functions of superego," "benign superego," "punitive superego," and "superego lacunae."

Superego lacunae, a popular term a few decades ago, refers to the deficit in the superego of persons who incompletely identify with their parents' critical and punishing aspects. It was assumed that when therapeutic work encountered a severe deficit or a hole in a patient's superego, the patient would act as though no work has been done in areas surrounding the lacuna. When we consider the superego as a collection of diverse compromise formations and an integration of various superego precursors, we believe that there is no need to speak of "superego lacunae." Some forms of superego functioning may be seen as clinically pathological, while others approach what we think of as "normal."

Latency phase

After dealing with the oedipal issues, a child enters the latency phase that extends until the onset of puberty. During this period, the child's energies from the sexual and aggressive drives are employed for nonsexual and nonaggressive interests in the outer world, beyond the family environment. The child finds new friends and teachers, improves his or her communication and social skills, becomes involved in sports or other extracurricular activities, and learns about rules and fairness. Selma Kramer and Joseph Rudolph (1980) wrote about "a sublimation of sexual curiosity into intellectual curiosity" (p. 111) during the latency phase. During this phase, there is also an internal struggle that is related to a wish to masturbate or the postponement of such a wish.

Genital phase and the adolescence passage

With the onset of puberty, a male becomes fully aware that the penis is not a part of the body used only for urination, and that semen also comes out from the penis. Girls' investment in their vagina increases as they become aware of the maturation of their breasts. Both boys' and girls' sexual as well as aggressive interests find new objects outside their family environment.

Anna Freud (1936, 1968) expanded her father's remarks about the genital phase by focusing on how physiological and endocrinological changes in the body reawaken the sexual and aggressive drives and the oedipal issues and internal conflicts during the adolescence passage. Going through an adolescent passage provides a model for adult-type mourning; a youngster reviews images of childhood, modifying some while discarding others and gaining new ones. (Also see: Blos, 1966, 1979; Wolfenstein, 1966, 1969.) Parents may recognize this type of mourning, for instance, when their older, college-age children wistfully reminisce about their childhood or derive bittersweet enjoyment from looking through photographs of their childhood years.

CHAPTER 7

Defense mechanisms

In 1936, Anna Freud began to offer a list of defense mechanisms. These defenses, appearing singly or occurring together, are used unconsciously to reduce anxiety. There are three basic types of anxiety: Reality Anxiety, which is a fear of a real danger in the external world, Neurotic Anxiety, which is a fear originating in the ego that it will not be able to control unconscious impulses (Eros and Thanatos), and Moral Anxiety, which is related to fear of retribution from the superego or conscience. To deal with these forms of anxiety, the ego uses a number of defense mechanisms.

Jerome Blackman (2004) named 101 types of defenses including repression, denial, reaction formation, splitting, rationalization, displacement, externalization, internalization, undoing, regression, etc. Defense mechanisms vary depending on a person's level of personality organization or level of psychopathology. The use of defense mechanisms is a normal function of the ego and is something everyone utilizes.

People without overt psychopathology use defense mechanisms like humor—where the expression of uncomfortable thoughts and feelings is made easier by making them funny, suppression—which is a conscious forgetting or putting something out of mind, and perhaps the healthiest defense mechanism, sublimation—which is a channeling of an unacceptable impulse into something acceptable. In fact, Freud (1930a) believed that human civilization has its origins in the sublimation of aggressive impulses into the creation of societal as well as physical structures.

Other more neurotic defense mechanisms include intellectualization—which is using intellectual processes to avoid experience of emotions, displacement—which is a shifting of unacceptable feelings toward one person onto another, and reaction formation—which is where an unacceptable feeling is transformed into its opposite.

More primitive defenses include splitting—which is the dissociation of feelings into all good or all bad, projection—which is the placement of feelings onto someone else, and dissociation—which is where a person separates themselves from an experience.

Defense mechanisms can also function as a form of resistance. If a defense is used to blunt therapeutic insight and to sabotage working-through, it can be understood as functioning as a resistance. Defense mechanisms working as resistances are typically related to transference and countertransference, as well as real-world aspects of the patient's relationship with the psychoanalyst or psychotherapist. A good example of a defense mechanism that is also a resistance is the so-called "flight into health." This is where a person comes to one or two therapy sessions but then suddenly is better and stops coming to therapy. In actuality, the person still has the issues that caused them to seek therapy in the first place.

CHAPTER 8

Resistances

In 1920, Sigmund Freud wrote that every step of treatment is accompanied by resistance. Patients resist involvement in a therapeutic process that will sabotage their mostly unconscious ways of dealing with their mental conflicts and the influence of their unconscious pathogenic fantasies. Resistance is not simply a reaction to the personality of a psychoanalytic clinician, although a clinician's personal issues and inexperience can contribute to the patient's resistance. Earlier in this book, for example, we describe how a young psychoanalyst, by placing a huge sword on the wall next to his couch, played a key role in his patient's resistance to deepening his analysis.

In 1926, Sigmund Freud referred to five types of resistance:

1. Repression resistance
2. Transference resistance
3. The gain of illness resistance
4. Repetition compulsion resistance, and
5. Superego resistance.

The first three types come from the ego, the fourth from the id, and the fifth from the superego (Freud, 1926d).

Freud (1937c) explored this subject further in "Analysis Terminable and Interminable," in which he distinguished resistances that reflect the ego's defensive operations from those built into the nature of the psychic apparatus that are etiologically independent of conflict. The latter include biological-constitutional factors, which Freud referred to as mobility of libido, loss of plasticity, adhesiveness of libido (in old age), and traumatic experiences. According to Freud, psychoanalysis takes a long time because of strong resistances. He acknowledged that sometimes a very intense and rigid resistance cannot be removed by psychoanalysis, leading to treatment failure.

Resistance in psychotherapy

What is true of psychoanalysis, in the case of resistance, is also true for psychoanalytic psychotherapy. Generally, psychoanalytic psychotherapy is considered a "long-term" psychotherapy. Glen Gabbard, in his excellent book *Long-Term Psychodynamic Psychotherapy* (2004), defines long-term psychotherapy as any psychotherapy that is more than twenty-four sessions or six months in duration. Although newer, shorter-term psychoanalytic therapies have been developed, these do not work with resistances in the same way. These shorter-term therapies utilize other aspects of psychoanalytic psychotherapy and are more focused on symptom reduction than personality change. In other words, they focus more on increasing the patient's ability to adapt his or her personality than to change it. There really is no shortcut to working with resistance in any kind of psychoanalytic treatment.

During the 1960s and 1970s, several so-called "humanistic" psychotherapies, a few of which were created by psychoanalysts, sought in essence to shortcut the process of working with defenses and resistances. This was done by having the psychotherapist take a much more directive role in the therapy, making suggestions and attempting to lead patients (now called clients) to insight.

Kevin Volkan has had a wide variety of experience (both as therapist and patient) with these psychodynamic but directive therapies, including Gestalt therapy (Perls et al., 1965), transactional analysis (Berne, 1961), and even primal scream therapy (Janov, 1970). In his experience, these therapies lead to some insight into defenses and resistance but rely, to varying degrees, on catharsis. After the cathartic release, the therapeutic insights gained seem to rapidly disappear or are repressed. The pressure from the repressed material then builds up, and under the direction of the therapist, the client then has another cathartic experience, along with temporary insight and relief. And so the cycle continues over and over. In many cases, what was supposed to be a shortcut and a short-term therapy drags on. Kevin Volkan has seen clients of these types of therapies remain with the same therapist for years and years, in a way addicted to the cycle of catharsis.

That is not to say that these therapies do not help clients adapt to their life circumstances, but in our opinion, true and permanent gain of insight is extremely rare. It is therefore not surprising that these forms of therapy have fallen out of favor and are now rarely taught to aspiring psychotherapists. The exception to these forms of therapy is so-called existential psychoanalysis (Boss, 1979) or existential psychotherapy (Yalom, 2009). This type of "humanistic psychotherapy" retains many of the qualities and techniques of psychoanalysis and does not seek a quick fix or focus on cathartic release. Likewise, the client-centered psychotherapy developed by Carl Rogers (1951) retains many psychodynamic aspects, though it does not use interpretation.

Some of the critique of humanistic psychotherapies can also be leveled at newer psychotherapies, such as cognitive-behavioral therapy, and its offshoots, such as acceptance-commitment therapy. However, the difference is that symptom reduction is the explicit goal of these therapies, and they do not make as much claim to permanent personality change. Because of this, these cognitive behavioral therapies may more easily partner with psychoanalytic therapies, with the cognitive behavioral therapies focusing on quick symptom reduction while allowing subsequent psychoanalytic psychotherapy to work for deeper adaptation or personality change.

Types of resistance

Repression resistance is utilized to avoid anxiety. As Karl Menninger (1958) wrote, "The ego has a habit ... to hold back certain things from expression, and this automatically extended to the analytic situation, especially when the expression of previous *repressed* impulses ...

becomes likely to occur" (p. 105). But patients, especially when they begin their psychoanalytic treatment, may also utilize other habitual ways of dealing with their internal problems in the sessions. We think that it would be more practical if we replace Freud's term "repression resistance" with the term "defense resistance" (V. D. Volkan, 2010). When a defense is used against insight and working-through, it also functions as a resistance. Patients' defense resistances will be influenced by the transference, countertransference, and the reality relationship with the psychoanalyst or the psychotherapist.

Transference resistance is derived from an expectation of "disappointment" in the psychoanalytic clinician. A patient expresses resistance in words or actions against the awareness of a more crucial issue. For example, a patient focuses on sexual expectations from the psychoanalytic clinician (or another individual representing the clinician) to hide his or her deprivation from a mothering person and to prevent working on this crucial element of his or her mental problems with the psychoanalytic clinician. This is illustrated in a case from Vamık Volkan's textbook on psychoanalytic treatment (2010):

Case example of transference resistance

Linda came to analysis after breaking off a stormy love affair with a married man, the fifth such affair in four years. As her psychoanalysis progressed, the origins of this behavior were revealed. During her oedipal phase of life, Linda's mother was depressed, drank heavily, and was hospitalized from time to time. At the time of her oedipal passage and later as a teenager, her father spoke of Linda as his "second wife," took her out without her mother, and treated her in such a way that she felt oedipal triumph.

In the second year of her psychoanalysis, Linda became infatuated with a professor at a university where I was also a professor; she filled her sessions with talk about him. After collecting enough information, I explained to her that the affair was a displacement of her feelings for me onto the professor, and, before long, the affair ended.

Linda then began to dress for her sessions with great care, became seductive on the couch, and declared her "love" for me. For months she spoke of nothing but her fantasized future with me. When I tried to connect her infatuation to the special relationship she had with her father as a child she could not hear it. Her psychoanalysis seemed to be at a standstill, although I maintained a psychoanalytic position and remained curious. When by chance Linda saw me at a theater with a woman, Linda protested angrily in the next session about this "rejection." However, this external event encouraged her use of reality testing, and, afterwards, more routine psychoanalytic work became possible.

In this case, Linda's difficulty acknowledging guilt about replacing her mother as her father's "second wife," and her fear of losing her mother's love in the process, made up primary sources of resistance. A very troubled and alcoholic mother could not provide good mothering for little Linda. As long as Linda preoccupied herself with her love for her father/lover/psychoanalyst, she could keep painful feelings associated with the depriving mother at bay. By developing an exaggerated *erotic transference*, Linda was maintaining her usual ways of handling mental conflict, steering clear of her wish to find a "good" mother and her dread that such a person might not exist. If the latter was true, she would be devastated and enraged. It was only after her very intense erotic transference development attenuated that the main source of this resistance came to the surface and could be truly understood and worked through. One of Kevin Volkan's psychoanalytic psychotherapy groups shows this.

Case example of erotic transference

During the course of group psychotherapy, a woman named Khloe developed what seemed to be an erotic transference toward me. This was in the context of a psychoanalytic psychotherapy group that consisted of seven women and a male and female therapist. During her second year of therapy, Khloe began to come to the group therapy sessions wearing revealing clothing and sit directly in front of me. I became curious about this behavior and felt it had something to do with Khloe's father. During the therapy sessions, Khloe was able to relate that her father often traveled for business and when he was home, paid little attention to her. Khloe was also married to a man who worked as a traveling salesman and who was often away from home, leaving Khloe to care for her two sons. After a while, Khloe would arrive for the group therapy sessions in her revealing outfits as before, only now clearly without a bra. As she would sit down in front of me, her nipples would become erect and stay this way for the therapy session. This continued for several weeks, even as Khloe began discussing how she felt about her father during her childhood.

I initially thought that Khloe's exaggerated erotic transference toward me was rooted in her early relationship with her distant father. However, some clues emerged that indicated Khloe's erotic transference might be a form of resistance. At one point, Khloe mentioned her sons and how she was worried that they might be unhealthy because they were not getting enough nourishment. When my female co-therapist tried to explore this with Khloe, she became angry and only wanted to speak with me. I asked if she was worried that she might be a bad mother. At this, Khloe became sad and began to cry. She then revealed that while her father was away, her mother would often go out at night to carouse, forgetting to feed Khloe and her siblings. Khloe's mother would dress in revealing outfits, especially low-cut clothing that showed her ample bosom. Khloe was now able to realize she carried a lot of anger toward her mother, who put her own pleasure ahead of taking care of her children. Her coming to the therapy sessions and displaying her nipples was her way of remembering her childhood mother as well as expressing her unconscious wish to be a good mother and nourish her children. After beginning to explore her relationship with her mother during the therapy sessions, Khloe's erotic behavior stopped, and she was able to make progress in therapy.

The gain of illness resistance takes place when a patient maintains his or her symptoms because they satisfy some internal demands or strivings. Through his or her symptoms, this patient receives gratification from the people or the situation in his or her environment.

Case example of illness resistance

Paul, a man in his mid-twenties, sought psychoanalytic psychotherapy because of having a feeling of not being able to move his right arm properly. He was informed by his orthopedic physician that his arm had no physical difficulty, but he was not able to give up his belief that he was a physically injured man. His physician suggested that Paul seek psychological help.

The following story came to the surface very early in Paul's treatment. Paul was working in his rich uncle's grocery store. He had an ambivalent relationship with his uncle, who owned the store and represented a father figure to him. Paul was anxiously engaged in conscious competition with the older man. He fantasized about making love to his uncle's secretary who, in Paul's mind, was his uncle's mistress.

One day he had an argument with his uncle and thought about hitting and kicking him. While he was in this angry mood, a heavy box fell on him, knocking him unconscious. Although his doctor reassured him that he had suffered no lasting physical damage, Paul continued to "suffer" from the blow he had sustained. His symptoms of pain and other accident-related complaints won him considerable attention from his uncle, while the secretary pampered him.

Paul's symptoms continued to exist for two and a half years. His frustrated family physician again urged him to seek psychological treatment: Paul's psychoanalytic psychotherapy revealed that he was resistant to giving up his symptoms since he received much gratification through them. They helped satisfy his punitive superego, since he perceived the blow from the box as punishment for the aggressive feelings he had harbored toward the uncle/father of his childhood, the source of much guilt. Staying "ill" kept him from knowing his death wishes toward his uncle/father. Moreover, his symptom won him a dependent position in which he got considerable attention from his uncle and the "forbidden woman," his uncle's secretary—all without fear of retaliation since, because of the accident, he was already damaged. After Paul became aware of the reason for his remaining as a bodily injured young man, he started perceiving his psychotherapist as a castrating oedipal father figure in the transference, and then slowly resolved his oedipal issues.

Repetition compulsion resistance refers to repeating traumatic events to try to gain mastery over them. Noting this compulsion to repeat, Freud (1920g) theorized about some demonic force opposing the pleasure principle and came to attribute repetition compulsion to mental operations more primitive in a biological-evolutionary sense than those normally directed by pleasure/displeasure. Accordingly, he developed his theory of the *death instinct* as opposed to the *life instinct*. (Later, such concepts were debated and for all practical purposes abandoned, and the death instinct is now thought of as instinctual aggression.)

Our focus here is on the role repetition plays in resistance during psychoanalysis as well as psychoanalytic psychotherapy. When viewed from this perspective, the tendency to repeat can be understood as a force opposing the patient's attempts to leave behind pathological patterns after their meanings are interpreted, understood, and owned. In the clinical setting, repetition compulsion is most clearly noticed when a childhood trauma and the patient's habitual response to it continue to repeat for some time after the patient learns and owns its meaning.

This is one of the most common patterns we see, though in addition to a resistance, the repetition can also be an attempt to gain mastery over a past situation. Sometimes the repetition can be related to anniversaries and other triggering events as well. One of Vamık Volkan's cases, which was mentioned in his (2010) textbook, demonstrates this principle.

Case example of repetition compulsion resistance

Cindy, a twenty-eight-year-old married social worker and mother of three small children, came to psychoanalysis with obsessional thoughts of harming her children by doing sexual things to them. Her symptom had appeared six months earlier, during a time she was looking after a young girl who had been sexually abused by her father. Cindy had herself been involved in an incestuous relationship with her own father from the age of eight until she reached puberty, at which time her father abruptly ceased having sexual intercourse with her for fear of making her pregnant.

When Cindy started psychoanalysis, she reported having complex feelings about her father. Both of her parents were still living. She said she had forgiven her father because he had been immature as a younger man and had always been kind to her. Her only negative feeling about him seemed to center on his abrupt rejection of her when she reached puberty. However, within a year of psychoanalysis, both Cindy and I became aware of Cindy's helplessness, humiliation, and rage over what had happened to her, and of her displacement of this rage onto her own children.

Cindy had a near-fatal accident in her early teens, and psycho-analysis revealed that she had experienced this as a punishment. Since she stubbornly clung to the mental image of this accident, she constantly put herself in a psychological position in which she paid for her "sins."

In many of her activities, Cindy symbolically repeated her sexual relationship with her father. For example, she had been a sexually promiscuous teenager, playing Russian roulette with the possibility of becoming pregnant. When she married in her late teens, she used her obsessional husband as an external superego against her impulses to act out sexually. However, her habit of bathing in the nude with her children without conscious concern about overstimulating them was a derivative of her relationship with her father.

During her marriage, her perception of herself as a flawed and marked woman played out incessantly. For example, despite her education, she never surrendered her country accent, only learning the meaning of this in psychoanalysis: her "bad accent" stood for her "bad sexuality"— incest. As a child, she had been mercilessly teased about her accent. Now, at professional meetings she arranged to have herself presented as "a country girl who made good," or as someone "with humble roots." Although this humiliated her, she insisted upon it—repetition compulsion was at work.

Cindy's associations made it clear that by repeatedly calling attention to her "faults," she was masochistically collecting witnesses for the sexual injustice done to her as a child. I was the first person to whom she talked about the incest. However, by parading her shortcomings, Cindy had symbolically been telling this story for some time. Other meanings, too, were condensed in these repetitions, which represented her fruit-less attempt to repeat her humiliation for the sake of mastering it and to maintain an attachment, even a painful and destructive one.

Once a piece of jewelry was stolen from Cindy's handbag, and she rushed to her father's house to get his sympathy for her loss. Instead, he blamed her for inviting the thief to steal her jewelry, saying, "It's your fault, *again*." She was filled with anger and frustration. I told her that the handbag represented her vagina and that she had experienced incestu-ous "rape" when she was robbed. I also said that her desire to "re-discuss" the theft with her father of today, who represented the father who had been involved with her sexually, was a way to "re-test" their relationship. She sought her father's sympathy and understanding but was left alone with her self-blame. My explanation helped her realize that she had felt confused, robbed, betrayed, angry, and guilty at the time of the incest. She had believed as a child that it was her fault. She cried her heart out in her next session and experienced much relief. Soon, however, she was ready to repeat her incestuous behavior in the transference. This time, her repetition compulsion was, in a sense, good for the therapeutic process, since reenacting the representation of a traumatic event between patient and psychoanalyst made the event authentic and available for working through.

At one point in the second year of her analysis, when Cindy left her psychoanalyst's office, she "forgot" her handbag. During her next therapeutic session, she fantasized that I, like the thief who stole her jewelry, went into, and explored the personal belongings in her handbag, her symbolic vagina. I refrained from quickly sharing with her my understanding that she was repeating in the transference the representation of her sexual relationship with her father. I wanted her to own her emotions. Thus, she stayed in a highly emotional state for several weeks, recalling symbolically and experiencing her sexual stimulation, her confusion, her rage, and her guilt. In the transference, Cindy slowly worked through the impact of her incest.

In her third year of psychoanalysis, Cindy seemed to have an improved sense of self and slowly began to lose her fear of harming her children, although her repetition compulsion did not completely disappear. She underwent an emergency appendectomy in her fourth year of analysis, and this recalled the psychology of rape as forceful penetration. In response, she again began to behave in an exaggerated way as a country bumpkin, a flawed woman. For some months, she repressed the meaning of her resumption of this symptomatic behavior. In her fifth year of psychoanalysis, she was a candidate for promotion at work and was required to take a written test. Her impulse to be a woman with a bad past, a country bumpkin, led her to make many embarrassing grammatical errors on the test; her repetition compulsion was resisting success in life and in treatment. She was not promoted at this time but did advance in her career just before ending psychoanalysis.

In routine analytic work, the intensity and duration of repetition compulsion attenuates over time with a gradual diminution of symptomatic patterns of affect, thought, and behavior. Psychoanalysis and psychoanalytic therapy afford patients an opportunity not only to repeat, but also to step outside of a pattern with the help of the psychoanalytic clinician, in order to identify and understand conflicts that drive a particular way of being. Through this process, repetition compulsion slowly loses its force and significance to the patient and, therefore, can be eventually given up.

The development of workable transference takes on the pattern of a repetition compulsion. Repetition of experiences in the psychoanalytic situation is beneficial as long as patients repeat their experiences, and they are helped to see and grasp their meanings. There is a chance for a "creative" repetition, wherein repeating creates the opportunity to review, reconsider, reflect, and repair. Thus, repetition has a role in working through.

Should we call repetition compulsion a resistance or should we accept it as an expected human trait that also appears in analysis? We feel that it is better not to refer to repetition compulsion only as a resistance. If the therapeutic work succeeds, what is repeated and troublesome for the patient starts shrinking. Our perception is that repetition compulsion never totally disappears, rather its duration shortens, and its influence is tamed.

Superego resistance can arise from a sense of guilt and, associated with this, a felt need for punishment according to the dictates of the superego. Freud (1941e) considered superego resistance to be the most obscure, although not always the weakest, of the five forms of resistance. It is present in almost every case, including the cases reported above. For example, Paul punished himself to keep his aggressive thoughts about his uncle/father unconscious. Cindy utilized her husband and the supervisors at her workplace as an external superego and experienced a near-fatal accident as a punishment stemming from her superego. The activation of the punishing forces of the superego acts as a resistance against gaining insights during the analytic process and against its deepening. One of Kevin Volkan's cases provides an illustration of this.

Case example of superego resistance

After approximately a year of once-a-week psychoanalytic psychotherapy, Adam was making good progress and had developed more insight into his internal world. Adam had been ordered by a court to obtain psychotherapy after he had been found guilty of unlawful touching of a minor. Abruptly, during a session, Adam asked me if I would write a letter to the court indicating that they should allow him to regain possession of his firearms. Adam was a gun collector and was required to give up his collection after his conviction. I immediately answered Adam with a hard no to this request. However, I was able to explore with Adam why he had made this request when he must have known it would be turned down. Over the next few weeks, Adam was able to articulate his anxiety that if he made good progress eventually I would terminate psychotherapy. By making me into a superego-like authority, Adam was working against his therapy. However, by interpreting and working through this resistance, Adam was ultimately able to make progress.

When a patient reports that he or she was tempted to steal something of significant value but refrained from doing so, we may assess to what extent the punitive aspects of his or her superego and aspects of his or her ego-ideal are integrated. The superego of an individual who refrains from stealing because of fear of punishment differs from that of another individual who does not steal because stealing would mean disappointing the expectation of this person's ego-ideal. If we are to speak about "superego" resistance, besides the expectation of punishment we should also take into consideration that patients may resist working in analysis if they unconsciously fear that psychoanalytic insight would threaten their ability to live up to their ego-ideal.

Object relations theory (Jacobson, 1964; Kernberg, 1976, 1988; V. D. Volkan, 1976, 1995) has removed the need to speak about "precursors" of superego and thus our need to utilize an adjective in front of the word "superego." Object relations theory informs us as to how one's libidinally and aggressively invested self and object images become integrated. Terms from object relations theory that refer to various types of unintegrated object images with associated affects that influence behavior provide better explanations of our patients in psychoanalytic treatment than does the term superego. It is clinically more helpful to explain the specific character of an internalized aspect of the punitive or idealized object images that interferes with the patient's gaining insight and working through mental conflicts.

Negative therapeutic reaction

The concept of *negative therapeutic reaction*, coined by Sigmund Freud (1923b) refers to a clinical phenomenon peculiar to the patient's psychology that is not susceptible to "routine" treatment and is thus unrelated to an analyst's mismanagement of the therapeutic relationship. Negative therapeutic reaction is the worsening of a patient's condition when everything in the psychoanalytic process calls for improvement and the relief of symptoms. In 1924, Freud indicated a "moral" factor and a sense of guilt in patients finding atonement in illness and refusing to give up the penalty of suffering. To some degree, the case of Adam, above, is representative of this.

Stanley Olinick (1980) states that in infancy and childhood some patients identify with a depressed pre-oedipal mother, and as adults experience their partners (in life or in the analytic dyad) variously as an internalized or externalized bad object—the depressed, devouring, but needed maternal image. Arthur Valenstein (1973) suggests that such patients may experience negative therapeutic reactions. Shelton Heath (1991) wrote that when a patient externalizes his or her depression on the psychoanalyst, the latter's task of staying in the therapeutic position may be taxing. Psychoanalytic clinicians' conscious—but more importantly, unconscious—thoughts and affects about the patient who frustrates them may cause further complications and make dealing with the negative therapeutic reaction quite difficult.

We suggest that a psychoanalytic clinician sensing such a reaction may benefit from consultation with another colleague to find out if there may be therapeutic ways to deal with it. This is especially true when the negative therapeutic reaction can engender countertransference. Because of this, and in general, we believe that consultation with an experienced colleague, as well as supervision for difficult cases, is underutilized and should become a more accepted part of the psycho-analytic therapeutic culture.

Resistance as part of "psychic surface"

Ella Freeman Sharpe (1950) listed rather typical personality traits that operate both in everyday life and in analysis as resistance. For example, some patients use charm, humor, thoughtfulness toward others, or extreme intellectualization to disarm the psychoanalyst or psychotherapist. Some of these characteristics function as defense mechanisms as well, and there can be difficulty in distinguishing their defensive versus resistive functions, since in both cases they protect the patient from anxiety.

Other patients exhibit resistance by becoming like obedient children. They are never late in coming to the therapy sessions and seem to accept every interpretation offered by the psychoanalyst or psychotherapist without actually benefiting from these interpretations. There are other patients who habitually control their psychoanalysts or psychotherapists by wondering aloud if he or she knows a particular thing: "I wonder if you read this book" or "… saw this movie." Sharpe warns us that a patient's overemphasized interest or affect might indicate a correspond-ing repressed one. For example, a patient presenting masochism may be defending his or her sadism.

Patients can also manifest resistance by giving their therapist a "gift." This can be an actual gift, or some other attempt to get the therapist to like the patient in an effort to control them. For example, during psycho-analytic psychotherapy, Kevin Volkan inadvertently found out that the psychoanalyst conducting his therapy was a Kleinian. Soon thereafter he started to have "shit" dreams that included feces in the content—something Melanie Klein famously found interesting. By giving her a "gift," his psychoanalyst could unconsciously be controlled. Once this was interpreted, the dreams stopped and psychotherapy progressed.

Activities as resistance

Patients can also use an activity for resistance. One patient of Vamık Volkan's, Thomas, used to cancel unacceptable thoughts and affects, reconstructions of his childhood, or interpretations of transferences through magical activities *in the analyst's office*. During one period of his treatment, Thomas would unconsciously make a downward gesture with his hand just before getting up from the couch. Slowly, it became evident that Thomas was "magically" flushing a toilet, as if therapeutic explanations or interpretations were fecal material to be flushed away. His magical gesture was a direct expression of his resistance.

Another case of Vamık Volkan's exemplifies how an activity *outside the analyst's office* can function as a resistance. It also exemplifies how resistance that includes an activity persists even after a patient has made great advances in analysis.

Case example of activity as resistance

As a child, Ralph was angry with his father, fantasized about mutilating him, and expected retaliation for these feelings. As a married man, he was prone to extreme castration anxiety. During his second year of psychoanalysis, he opened his session one Monday afternoon by saying that he had bought a paperweight two days before. As he described its shape, it seemed that it resembled a phallus.

The weekend he bought the paperweight, he touched it often, and when he left home without it on Monday, he felt uneasy. He thought that he might take it to his office and use it as a dumbbell to help him lose weight and get in shape. After speaking about the paperweight, Ralph focused on his weight gain and talked about how his distended abdomen made his penis look smaller. Listening to Ralph, I thought, "The patient bought a symbolic penis. His wish to use it as a dumbbell seemed to promise not only a loss of weight, but also an attendant enhancement of his penis size."

Soon Ralph revealed that his father had been admitted for a cataract operation and that he had bought the paperweight right after seeing his father's eyes bandaged. This was reminiscent of how Oedipus blinded himself in an act of self-castration after learning that he had killed his father and married his mother. Since Ralph was in his second year of psychoanalysis and was already aware of his castration anxiety, I explained to him that the sight of his father symbolically castrated (by the eye operation) had made Ralph anxious lest he, in turn, be castrated.

I continued: "Remember your telling me last week about buying a big car. Remember also comparing your new car's size with the size of my 'old junk' when you parked your new car next to mine. [My car was parked in front of the building where I had my office and Ralph had referred to it in a previous session as an 'old junk.'] You were so happy. I noticed your big smile. But then you became so fidgety. Remember how we talked about your putting your hands in your trouser pockets and checking on your penis. Remember my saying 'It is still there,' and you bursting into laughter. I thought it was good: you could have a penis and I could have one too. Why not? We could compare their sizes for a while. Then you went to the hospital and noticed that a doctor 'blinded' your father, that big guy. I remember your telling me way back how you had a dream on your early teens and in this dream your father was blinded. Now that your childhood dream came true, what will be your fate? OK, you bought an extra phallus, the paperweight, in case you lose your real penis." Ralph burst into laughter again and was relieved by my explanation of his resistance. After this session, he no longer invested the paperweight with any magical property.

Built-in transference

Some patients start their psychoanalytically oriented treatments after seeing another therapist for some time and developing strong transference feelings toward, and expectations from, the previous therapist. These patients might have experienced different therapeutic approaches while working with their previous therapists. As these patients enter a new treatment, it is likely that they will carry what can be called a *built-in transference*. That is, this person may unconsciously relate to the present psychoanalytic clinician as an extension of, and thus not clearly separate from, past therapists, even if the capacity to distinguish between them intellectually is intact. Built-in transference can be utilized as a resistance. Noticing built-in transference and dealing with it helps a psychoanalytic psychotherapist to separate his or her therapeutic identity from the identity of the patient's previous therapists (V. D. Volkan, 2010; V. D. Volkan et al., 2002; Werman, 1984).

Case example of built-in transference

Denzel was twenty-three years old when he started to see a female psychotherapist twice a week, stating that he was feeling fidgety and frustrated. He was living in a small apartment by himself with financial support from his parents. He was not able to keep a steady job and his parents also paid for his treatment. The psychotherapist heard stories of Denzel's traumatic childhood. Denzel's father would beat him often and his mother would not protect him. Denzel had no siblings. As he grew up, he became aware of his repeating fantasy of wishing his parents to die in a car accident so that he could get their money.

After seeing Denzel for sixty-eight weeks, the psychotherapist felt that she needed support because she could not build a trusting relationship with this "very difficult patient" and asked for supervision. It emerged that Denzel had previously seen another female psychotherapist for 100 sessions on a twice weekly basis. He felt that his first therapist was like his mother, who could not protect and love him when he was a child. Denzel informed his new psychotherapist that while seeing his first therapist he had started killing cats. Whenever he saw and caught a cat, he would kill the *animal* that represented his first psychotherapist as a bad parent figure and throw away the dead animal in a trash can. He had never shared this information with his first therapist and impulsively left her ("killed" her).

Without examining and understanding Denzel's murderous transference wishes for his first psychotherapist it would be difficult for Denzel and his second psychotherapist to develop a working alliance and therapeutic relationship. Appropriately, the second psychotherapist softly told Denzel that they would be able to develop a working alliance when he put his feelings, however strong they may be, in words instead of expressing them by actions. The psychotherapist added that if Denzel killed another cat, she would stop seeing him. Denzel agreed.

Transference dilution

Something that is somewhat the opposite of built-in transference can also occur. This happens when a patient will see more than one therapist or therapy figure simultaneously. This type of resistance is common in places where psychotherapy specifically is culturally accepted, and wildly varying ideas about therapy are in common use. If this occurs, the transference to the primary psychoanalytic clinician does not get a chance to deepen. The patient then can keep the good and bad transference "split" among different therapists without having to gain the ability to see the therapist ambivalently as both good and bad.

We have also seen this among patients suffering from borderline personality disorder. A patient being treated by Vamık Volkan provides an example of this.

Case example of transference dilution

A patient, Joe, started seeing another therapist without informing me. In this case, having multiple therapists was connected to Joe's splitting of self and object images that were being addressed by me at this point in psychoanalysis. This induced a good deal of resistance. I told Joe that if he kept me as a "half-therapist" I could not help him. I said to him I would continue to see him when he accepted me as "one person." Joe stopped his other "treatment" and continued to work with me.

There are some instances when having multiple therapy figures may be beneficial. Noted psychoanalyst Leon Wurmser, who worked with drug-addicted patients, encouraged many to enroll in Narcotics Anonymous. For Wurmser, this pseudo-therapy group functioned as an auxiliary superego that he thought beneficial to his drug-addicted patients (K. Volkan, 1994b). In one case report from Spain involving a psychotic male, multiple transferences with different clinicians was thought to be beneficial (de Angel & Turek, 1990).

Last words about resistance

We choose to continue to utilize the term resistance, although we consider it an expected and "normal" phenomenon. It is included—like symptoms, inhibitions, personality traits, and adaptations—in a patient's way of dealing with mental conflicts. Dealing with resistances is required, not only at the beginning phase but also throughout the treatment. Resistance is not a patient's deliberate attempt to struggle with the therapist. Psychoanalytic clinicians need to deal with resistance with empathy and respect, keeping a watchful eye on their own countertransference.

CHAPTER 9

Making formulations, interpretations, and working through

Now let us examine how a psychoanalytic psychotherapist might create a therapeutic foundation and environment during the initial phase of the treatment of an adult individual. Above we described how a psychoanalytic clinician's office and everything within it is a psychological extension of the clinician, along with how it should be designed. Regardless of whether the clinician is a psychoanalyst or psychoanalytic psychotherapist, it is important to borrow certain technical concepts from psychoanalysis when starting to work with a patient and setting up a therapeutic foundation and environment.

Setting up a psychotherapeutic environment

After completing diagnostic interviews, a psychoanalytic clinician who decides to conduct analysis or psychotherapy with an individual informs the new patient how the therapy sessions will be conducted: The patient will tell whatever comes to his or her mind and the therapist will talk whenever he or she thinks it will be useful. Karl Menninger (1958) wrote that a psychoanalyst "cannot promise cure; he cannot even promise relief. She or he can only promise to try to help the patient by a method that has helped others and on the condition that the patient try to help himself" (p. 31). Psychoanalytic clinicians also need to keep

Menninger's remarks in mind and bring to the patient's attention the importance of a "therapeutic alliance" (C. Brenner, 1979; Zetzel, 1956), which is a reality-based collaboration between the therapist and the patient that includes trust and ethics.

In psychoanalysis, it is typical for the patient to have four to five sessions a week. For psychoanalytic psychotherapists, we suggest that, when financially and realistically possible for the patient, it will be beneficial to see the patent at least twice a week instead of once a week. However, we realize that this is often not possible. Nevertheless, working with a patient who comes in no more than once a week does not change the use of psychoanalytic technique and strategy.

It has become increasingly common that a patient comes to a psycho-therapist for a very limited number of sessions seeking symptom relief. The psychotherapist might even employ non-psychoanalytic techniques. However, at the end of these sessions, the patient can be informed that a more permanent resolution of the issues underlying the symptoms can be sought with more long-term therapy. Some patients will want to continue therapy, at which time the milieu of psychoanalytic treatment can be discussed as well as frequency of sessions, etc. This integrated approach is now being used for a number of mental health issues including more severe mental illnesses (Berger, 2016; DiGiorgio et al., 2004; Garrett, 2019; Hauke et al., 2019; Leonidaki, 2021; Rudenstine et al., 2018; Schultz-Venrath et al., 2012; Shanok, 2015). It should also be noted that psychoanalytic concepts and principles are also being integrated into non-psychodynamic forms of psychotherapy (Wakefield & Baer, 2010).

The patient will be told to keep all of his or her appointments. Other practical issues such as payment for the sessions as well as payment for missing hours will also be explained. Psychoanalytic clinicians should pay particular attention to unconscious symbolic meanings and acting-out related to payment. This is one of the reasons that many psycho-analytic clinicians used to ask their patients to make payment after each session. In the modern world, this is no longer typical—the clinician might work for an agency, or in a hospital or university setting where payment is made to the institution. Or for business purposes, it may be better for the clinician to bill the patient once a month. However, if possible, exploration of unconscious meaning, transference manifestations (especially negative transference, as there is often anger around making payment), and resistance related to payment will reveal a great deal to the therapist. The legal constraints on confidentiality will be disclosed verbally and/or in writing. As discussed above, if the legal constraints on confidentiality become an issue at some point and the psychoanalytic clinician is required to break confidentiality, this will also likely evoke transference manifestations.

What am I treating? Psychodynamic case formulation

A psychoanalytic clinician's assessment of a patient's psychological makeup is known as a "formulation." After meeting a new patient, the psychoanalytic clinician wonders about what aspect of the patient's personality the clinician will be treating. A diagnosis is made about the patient's ego and superego functions, fixation on the developmental ladder level, and other defense mechanisms (A. Freud et al., 1965). Today, making a formulation also includes considerations about the nature of the patient's self-representation and object relationships, as well as his or her responses to traumas experienced not only in childhood but also in adulthood. Additionally, the psychoanalytic clinician will be attentive to the intertwining of external and internal events and possibilities for the nature of transference developments and possible counterresponses (McWilliams, 1999; V. D. Volkan, 2010).

To make a satisfactory case formulation, the clinician needs to collect enough data about the patient's developmental history. An initial case formulation prepares the clinician not only intellectually, but also emotionally, to conduct the treatment. As psychoanalysis or psychoanalytic psychotherapy progresses and new observations and data become available, some changes or additions to the initial case formulation may be required.

An example of an initial case formulation

Case example

A businessman named Andrew was fifty years old when he sought treatment. During his first face-to-face meeting with his psychotherapist, Andrew described why he sought treatment. He said that he was married for the second time and having unexpected rage attacks; he would break plates in the dining room, scream, and then go out for fresh air to calm down. He never had such temper tantrums during his first marriage. He was puzzled and feeling guilty. He wanted to understand what was happening to him and to rid himself of his disturbing symptoms.

Andrew went on to say that his first marriage was to a woman his age when he was thirty years old. The couple had no children, and he had no passion for his wife. He had known his second wife for a long time since she grew up in his neighborhood. She was twenty-two years younger than Andrew, who first used to think of her as his daughter. However, as she grew up, Andrew had sexual thoughts about her. When he was forty-eight years old, he began to have sex with the young woman, quickly divorced his wife, and married her. His symptoms began soon after.

During Andrew's initial two meetings with his psychotherapist, the following information became available. Andrew's father was a very rich businessman. He was distant from his son, who was his only child. His excuse was his preoccupation with his work. When Andrew's father reached the age of forty-eight, he developed cancer and died a few months after his illness was diagnosed. On his deathbed, he called his son, who was then twenty-two years old, and told him the following: "I had a huge business. I was like a king. I am now leaving my business, my kingdom, to you. Now you will be the king and take care of your mother."

After his father died, Andrew indeed became a very rich "king" at the age of twenty-two. His mother, who then was in her mid-forties, soon found a boyfriend. Interestingly, this boyfriend was the *same age* as her son. She told Andrew that her relationship with the young boyfriend was a platonic one; they were not having sex.

During his third diagnostic interview, Andrew began the session talking about his mother when he was a child. He described how his father went on frequent business trips and while he was away, his mother would often get drunk. One day, when Andrew was a pubertal child, he found his almost naked mother passed out in the living room with a bottle of bourbon next to her. He went on to describe in a matter-of-fact way and without much affect how he carried his mother to the parental bed. He added that he was embarrassed at that time because he had an erection after touching his mother's almost naked body.

Obviously, during these three fifty-minute sessions, Andrew spoke about other things as well.

Here, we are reporting data from Andrew's first three sessions to construct Andrew's psychological condition. Now we ask the reader to join us in making a formulation.

Let us begin with the information about Andrew's divorcing his first wife and marrying, at age forty-eight, a twenty-two-year-old woman whom he previously had considered as his "daughter." Did a psychological urgency that aimed to repeat, and perhaps to master, a past traumatic experience motivate this action? We can imagine that when his father died at age forty-eight, the patient replaced him as the "king"; in a sense, he had an oedipal triumph. By choosing a twenty-two-year-old boyfriend (a displacement figure for her son), Andrew's mother actively stimulated her son's mental conflict over having suddenly reached such a triumph. Perhaps, to deal with her own guilt feelings, the mother presented her relationship with the young man as platonic. (At this time, the psychotherapist did not know if Andrew believed his mother on a conscious level.)

Now we can develop a case formulation: When Andrew turned forty-eight years old, he reversed the "mother–son" incestuous intimacy with a "father–daughter" incestuous intimacy that included actual sexual activities. This broke the incest taboo, and increased Andrew's feelings of guilt and competition with other men. Andrew stated that he was afraid his wife would betray him with other men. He responded to such conflicts with angry outbursts.

Since age twenty-two (and perhaps since childhood), Andrew was fixated on concerns about sexuality and passion; something in him inhibited his expressing himself freely when he was with a woman. Andrew could not be a passionate man with his first wife while he was busy with such concerns. The psychotherapist noticed that while Andrew had a memory of having an erection when touching his mother's partially naked body, he used an isolation mechanism to deal with its ramifications. Andrew had no affects connected with the memory.

His young second wife belonged to another race. This itself might provide a defense mechanism: a woman whose race is different from his mother's race would "fool" Andrew's unconscious mind, since it would be impossible to think of the second wife as representing Andrew's mother.

Andrew had good reality testing and the ability to keep his father's business alive and healthy. The psychotherapist concluded that if he took Andrew into treatment, transference-countertransference manifestations primarily would center on resolving Andrew's oedipal struggle. Of course, the psychotherapist was aware that once treatment started, he and the patient most likely would also notice other psychological complications.

The psychotherapist had another thought: If Andrew resolved his conflicts, his second marriage (an expression of his oedipal conflict) might dissolve. On the other hand, the psychotherapist was aware of Andrew's pain. He also thought that if Andrew did not go through with psychoanalytic psychotherapy, his second marriage might still end, perhaps sooner, because of his angry outbursts and jealousy. The psychotherapist concluded that his task would be treating Andrew and that what Andrew and his second wife did with their marriage would be up to them. He offered psychoanalytic treatment to Andrew, who accepted this offer.

Preparatory and linking interpretations

The concept of interpretation describes a psychoanalytic clinician's verbalization of his or her understanding of what lies behind the patient's repeating behavior patterns, new events, disturbing relationships, dreams, daydreams, and so on. An interpretation aims to show the patient how his or her mind is working. When the psychoanalytic movement first began, it was claimed that cure is possible if the patient is made aware of repressed mental contents that are troublesome (Freud, 1895d). Such interpretations lead to a catharsis. It was Freud's important discovery that interpretation and its attendant catharsis alone do not result in a cure, and that interpretation must be repeated in order to allow the patient to internalize the clinician's understanding of the patient's psychic processes. Now we know that interpretation makes up only one aspect of the complicated processes that lead to internal structural changes in a patient. In today's psychoanalytic literature, we notice descriptions of different types of interpretations, such as resistance interpretations, content interpretations that describe genetic aspects of the patient's mental issues, and transference interpretations (Arlow, 1979; Levy, 1984).

Here we will focus on the initial phase of psychoanalytic treatment and describe *preparatory and linking interpretations*. The aim of a psychoanalytic clinician's initial communications is to prepare the patient to be curious about his or her internal psychological processes. In other words, these early communications are intended to help the patient develop an analytic mindset.

Rudolph Loewenstein (1951, 1958) described preparatory interpretations during the beginning phase of a treatment. Preparatory interpretations primarily focus on how something in a patient's internal world stimulates expected behavior in certain circumstances. The psychoanalytic clinician names the internal phenomenon without an in-depth description of what might have caused it. For example, the clinician notices that a male patient consistently tries to avoid competition with other male individuals. The clinician then verbalizes that the patient may be bound in unconscious rivalry that is demonstrated by his avoidance of competition. By stating that the patient's external behavior is due to an internal motive, the psychoanalytic clinician awakens the patient's curiosity about his or her internal world and helps the patient to explore his or her unconscious rivalry.

Peter Giovacchini (1969, 1972) first described linking interpretation, and this concept was later expanded further (V. D. Volkan, 1976, 1987). Giovacchini based his description of linking interpretation on Freud's (1900a) concept of *day residue* in dreams. Day residue is simply the appearance of events in the life of a person in his or her dreams after the event has occurred. It can be thought of an individual's memory traces of life events that stimulate dream content. The existence of day residue has been validated by empirical research (Veloce et al., 2019). Giovacchini applied Freud's understanding of day residue to the clinical setting, stating, "An interpretation may make a causal connection by referring to the day residue that may be the stimulus for the flow of the patient's associations or for some otherwise unexplainable behavior" (1969, p. 180).

Here are some examples of simple linking interpretation. The first case is Vamık Volkan's, and the second one is a case reported by the psychotherapist Volkan was supervising.

Case example of linking interpretation 1

While on the couch, a female patient looked at the ceiling and said that blood was dripping from holes in the ceiling tiles. I connected this bizarre perception with the patient's earlier statement that she had just begun menstruating, thus linking her identification of her bleeding body with a "bleeding" environment. At this phase of her treatment, this patient had begun to recall troublesome adolescence memories linked to the time when she started to menstruate.

Case example of linking interpretation 2

In his first psychotherapy session, Jimmy, a university student, described how he had an unusual feeling while driving to his psycho-therapist's office. He had an idea that something was wrong with one of his car tires. So, he pulled the car in at a safe place, got out, and inspected all four tires. They seemed intact. He resumed driving, but within minutes he was once more convinced that one of the tires had gone flat. Again, he stopped the car and checked all the tires, which were just fine. Nevertheless, when he parked his car in front of the psychotherapist's office, he once more had the impulse to check the tires. As before, the tires were sound. The psychotherapist had no idea why the patient had this unusual experience. Toward the end of the session, Jimmy reported that he had taken a four-part exami-nation. Although he was confident about three of the four parts, he thought he had done poorly in the fourth and feared failure. As he got into his car to drive to the psychotherapist's office, he thought that telling his psychotherapist about his possible failure in the exam-ination would embarrass him. Upon hearing this, the psychotherapist told the patient that his conviction that there were three good tires on his car might represent the three sections of the examination in which he had done well, while the imagined bad tire represented the section in which Jimmy performed poorly.

Working through

The aim of preparatory and linking interpretations is to help the patient to be ready to gradually receive "deep interpretations" as the treatment progresses, such as resistance interpretation, transference interpretations, as well as the deeper interpretation of the content of the patient's internal world and the patient's pathological ways of handling his or her mental conflicts. Such interpretations prepare the patient to be involved in what is known in the literature as "working through, the crucial part of psychoanalytic treatment." This term "working through" was coined first by Sigmund Freud (1914g). It refers to insights gained by deep

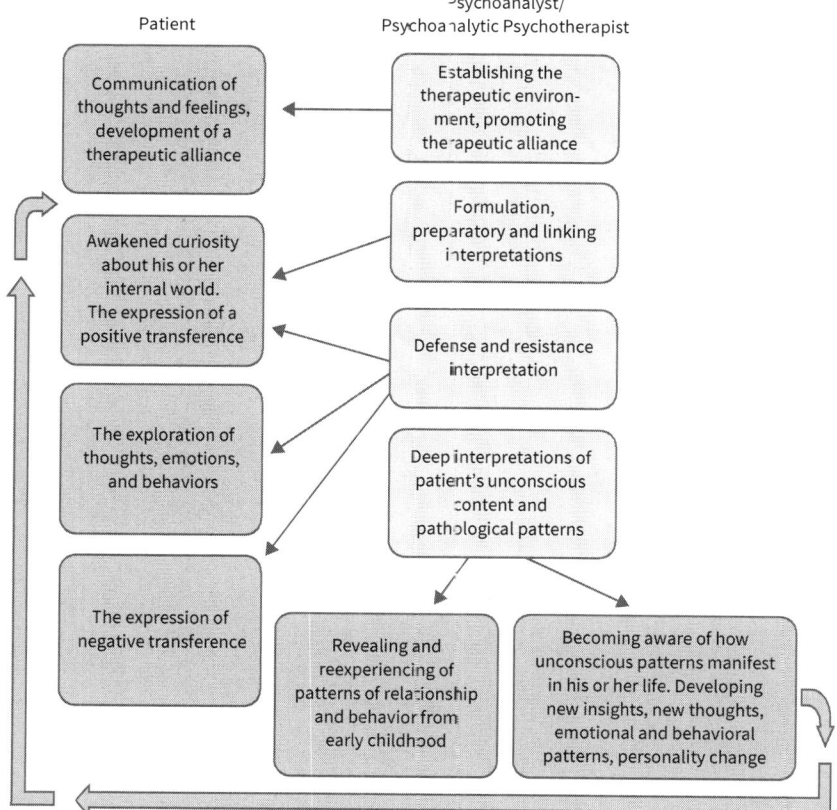

Figure 1 The working through process of psychoanalysis or psychoanalytic psychotherapy

interpretations making lasting positive changes in the patient, primarily due to altering how instinctual drives express themselves and by evolving new and better psychic adjustment to internal and external events (Loewald, 1988; Rycroft, 1972).

The process of working through is not a one-off. The working through process of psychoanalysis or psychoanalytic psychotherapy roughly follows this progression:

This therapeutic process of working through must be repeated.

CHAPTER 10

The separation–individuation level and psychosocial development

> my
> mother
> was
> my first country.
> the first place i ever lived.

—Nayyirah Waheed (2013, p. 212)

Sigmund Freud's description of psychosexual development was based on observations from the analysis of adults. Anna Freud, with Dorothy Burlingham (1942), observed babies and children during World War II in England and noted how anxiety passes from a mother or caregiver to the child. They noted that if mothers or caregivers remained calm during the German Luftwaffe bombings of London in World War II, the children did not become anxious. Conversely, when the children sensed anxiety in their mothers or caregivers, they too experienced anxiety. Direct observations of babies and children were later conducted by other psychoanalysts.

René Spitz (1965) illustrated that at about eight months of age, a baby develops the ability to differentiate his or her mother from strangers, and described the emergence of "separation anxiety." He also observed "social referencing,"—a child looking at his or her caregivers to check how they respond to something new. Donald Winnicott (1965, 1992) observed how an individual may develop a "false self" when he or she does not receive the required care and help from a "good-enough mother." Such an individual as an adult may be a success in the real world, but deep down he or she feels unsatisfied. John Bowlby (1958, 1960) wrote about babies' and children's "attachment." They need to develop a necessary relationship with at least one important person in their lives for normal emotional and social development. (For other examples, see: Emde, 1988a, 1988b, 1991; Fonagy & Target, 1997, 1998; Greenspan, 1997; Lehtonen, 2003; Parens, 2007). The realization that the development of a child's mind results from his and her interactions with mother or caregiver led Margaret Mahler (1958, 1968) to offer a new developmental ladder.

Mahler's theory of development

Normal autistic phase

Margaret Mahler's (1958, 1968) first stage, termed the normal autistic phase, characterizes the period from birth to ten or twelve weeks of age, when an infant is self-absorbed and does not have a sense that satisfaction of his or her needs comes from external sources. When new findings illustrated that a newborn infant's mind is more active than was previously thought, this phase was re-termed the "quasi-autistic phase" (Harley &Weil, 1979, p. xiii). Please note that the use of the term "autistic" here does not have the same meaning as the diagnosis of autism spectrum disorders.

Normal symbiotic phase

The normal symbiotic phase starts during the last part of the quasi-autistic phase and lasts until four or five months old. The infant is merged with the mother and does not have a separate sense of individuality.

Separation–individuation phase

Margaret Mahler (1968) divided a child's moving out of a symbiotic dual unity with his mother into four subphases of a separation-individuation phase:

Differentiation subphase

This first subphase exists from about four or five to nine or ten months, during which time the infant's awareness of the mother, and in general, the world, keeps increasing.

Practicing subphase

From nine or ten to fifteen or sixteen months, with his or her increased psychomotor ability, the infant experiences physical separations from his or her primary objects, the mother, or other mothering persons. But the infant also needs emotional refueling by running back to the primary object and touching her before experiencing another physical separation.

Rapprochement subphase

From fifteen or sixteen months to twenty-four months, the baby learns that he or she cannot control the mother. Separation anxiety surfaces, and the child experiences ambivalence, helplessness, and temper tantrums.

Object constancy

Successful completion of the rapprochement subphase marks the development of a steady internal mental image of important objects, such as the image of the mother. When the child is not physically near the mother, the child experiences an intrapsychic image of the mother. This process is accompanied by the child's development of a more realistic self-representation, one that is not fused with an intrapsychic image of the mother.

Second individuation

Peter Blos (1966, 1979) referred to the second individuation during *the adolescence passage*, the first individuation having been completed toward the end of the third year of life when children develop object constancy. In normal development, the natural regression that takes place during adolescence ushers in a new psychic organization. Both male and female youngsters review images of their childhood, modifying some while discarding others and accommodating new identifications. They develop more realistic knowledge about their own sexuality as well as the realistic and ethical issues they face.

We consider Jerome Blackman and Kathleen Dring's recent book, *Psychodynamic Developmental History and Evaluation of Children: Infancy to Adolescence* (2022), to be a valuable handbook for mental health workers, parents, grandparents, childcare workers, teachers, coaches, and anyone involved with children and adolescents. It includes questions about, and answers to, psychological issues during the child's developmental years.

Psychosocial development through a lifetime

Erik Erikson (1950, 1959, 1968) introduced eight steps of psychological development throughout a person's life and focused on struggles the individual faces at each step.

1. Trust vs. mistrust

From birth to eighteen months, an infant is totally dependent on the mother or caregiver for basic needs, such as food and comfort. When the infant's needs are not met, he or she will experience mistrust and fear.

2. Autonomy vs. shame and doubt

This phase lasts from eighteen months to three years old. A child at this stage starts learning about independence and how to control his or her body (such as while going through toilet training). If there is interference with the child's efforts in autonomy, this individual may develop self-doubt and shame.

3. Initiative vs. guilt

This phase takes place during pre-school years, from age three to age five. At this stage, the child finds new playmates, asks questions, and explores a wider world. If parents interfere with the child's activities, a sense of isolation, guilt and/or a lack of ambition will develop.

4. Industry vs. inferiority

From age five to twelve years, the child is in elementary school. Now he or she has teachers and new friends from different family backgrounds. Intellectual activities, such as learning mathematics, take place. The child becomes aware of his or her identity. However, if there are interventions, such as negative experiences at home, the child may experience society as too demanding and may develop role confusion.

5. Identity vs. confusion

During this period of psychosocial development, from age twelve to eighteen, the individual faces questions such as: "What is happening to my body?", "Who am I?", "What is my identity?", "How do I fit in to society?", and "What are my goals?" If there are no complications, the young person develops a strong sense of self and has a clear view of his or her future. But complications such as parents not allowing their offspring to find their own values and beliefs can also occur. This causes the teenager to experience confusion and/or insecurity.

6. Intimacy vs. isolation

Adulthood, from age nineteen to forty, is the time for a person to invest in commitment to others and build long-term loving relationships. If an individual could not develop a steady identity during the previous steps of psychosocial development, he or she will have difficulties in staying in committed relationships, and the individual will experience isolation, loneliness, and/or depression.

7. Generativity vs. stagnation

Between age forty and sixty-five, a person is busy with his or her family, the future of his or her children, careers, community affairs, charities, and/or societal events. The person is recognized by others as a productive member of society. However, perceived failure in usefulness and/or a perceived lack of accomplishments can cause the individual to experience stagnation and/or depression.

8. Integrity vs. despair

After age sixty-five, individuals look back and wonder what they have achieved. Some feel satisfied and proud. Others consider themselves to have been unproductive and this may lead to their experiencing depressive feelings. Erikson noted that at this late stage of life some individuals experience alternate feelings of satisfaction and regret.

A ninth step

After Erik Erikson died in 1994, his wife Joan added a ninth step to her husband's developmental ladder (Brown & Lowis, 2003). She referred to people in their eighties and nineties who are facing their own death and who experience the loss of some bodily and mental functions, the loss of some ability to move around, isolation from what is happening in the environment, and the loss of family members or friends. Joan Erikson suggested that people in their eighties and nineties may experience the trust vs. mistrust issues like a newborn baby in stage one. Or they find new skills such as play, activity, and song, and move beyond fear of death. They may be living in retirement communities or assisted living facilities.

Referring to retirement communities and assisted living facilities reminds us that the descriptions of developmental ladders offered by Joan Erikson, her husband, Margaret Mahler, and Sigmund Freud were all based on observations of children and adults in developed countries. We need to consider how societal, cultural, political, and economic issues influence a person's mind. We will give examples of this later in this book.

Individual identity and large-group identity

Surprisingly, Sigmund Freud used the word "identity" only five times in his writings. His well-known reference to identity is found in a speech he wrote that was delivered on his behalf at B'nai B'rith (a Jewish religious organization). In this paper, Freud wondered why he was bound to Jewry since, as a non-believer, he had never been instilled with ethno-national pride or religious faith. Nevertheless, Freud noted a "safe privacy of a common mental construction" and a clear consciousness of his "inner identity" as a Jewish individual (Freud, 1941e, p. 274).

It is interesting that Freud's remarks linked his individual identity with his large-group identity. Our term "large-group identity" refers to the thousands or millions of people, most of whom will never see or even know about each other as individuals, that share many of the same sentiments.

Identity was not originally considered a psychoanalytic term. Erik Erikson (1950, 1956, 1959), besides exploring societal and cultural influences on child development and defining the psychology of eight stages of human life, made the concept of personal "identity"— a subjective and persistent sense of sameness—an area of psychoanalytic inquiry. Erikson also showed interest in large-group identity.

He defined how at the outset of human history, each human group developed a distinct sense of identity, wearing skins and feathers like armor to protect it from other groups who wore different kinds of skins and feathers. Erikson hypothesized that each group became convinced that it was the sole possessor of the true human identity. Thus, each group also became a *pseudo species*, adopting an attitude of superiority over other groups.

Vamık Volkan became involved in international relations at the end of the 1970s as a member and then chairperson of the American Psychiatric Association's Committee on Psychiatry and Foreign Affairs during a six-year period of unofficial diplomatic talks by bringing together influential Israelis, Egyptians, and later, Palestinians. Subsequently, with a multidisciplinary team from the University of Virginia, Volkan brought together unofficial representatives of other opposing large groups, such as Americans-Soviets, Russians-Lithuanians, Russians-Estonians, Georgians-South Ossetians, Croats-Serbs, and Turks-Greeks for years-long series of talks aimed at mutual understanding and a more peaceful coexistence (V. D. Volkan, 1988, 1997, 2004, 2006b, 2013, 2020). During this work, the subjective experiences of such large-group identities were being expressed in terms such as, "We are Palestinians," "We are Lithuanian Jews," "We are Russians living in Estonia," "We are Croats," "We are Communists," and "We are Sunni Muslims."

"Group psychology" and the tent metaphor

Now we will briefly summarize Sigmund Freud's "group psychology" and then add new perspectives on his ideas. Freud did not consider mere collections of people to be a group, and described race, nations, and religious or professional organizations as groups. He illustrated that despite the differences between the Church and the army, each has a head (Jesus Christ, and a commander-in-chief) who rules and treats all individuals with equal love. In turn, the members idealize the leader, "put one and the same object in the place of their ego ideal" and identify "themselves with one another in their ego" (Freud, 1921c, p. 116). Freud linked the image of the leader to a "primal father" of a "primal horde" of prehistoric times (Freud, 1912–13), which has never actually been observed. Such a father prevents his sons from satisfying their sexual impulses. Only the father's successor will have the possibility of sexual satisfaction.

Freud also wrote how individuals in a large group develop new experiences such as losing distinctiveness and being subjective to suggestions. If mutual ties between the members cease to exist, panic starts. Freud also pointed out how belonging to a large group creates prejudice toward strangers. It was Robert Waelder (1936) who first stated that Freud was describing regressed large groups. (In Chapters 20 and 21, when we write about psychoanalytic concepts related to organizations and group psychotherapy, we will return to Freud's group psychology and further examine these concepts.)

Reading Freud's ideas about large-group psychology is reminiscent of the May Day or maypole dance, a tradition that goes back centuries and is related to the fertility of the harvest. Dancers, often holding ribbons, circle around a tall pole. The pole's symbolism has been mentioned by various scholars from different fields. Thinking of Freud's description of large-group psychology, let us consider the pole as representing the primal father. We have expanded the picture of the maypole dance by imagining a canvas extending from a tall pole out over all the people, forming a huge tent (V. D. Volkan, 1988, 2020). It is possible to also imagine how we learn to wear two layers, like fabric, from the time we are children. The first layer, the individual layer, fits each of us snugly, like clothing. It is a person's core individual identity. The second layer, the canvas of the tent, is shared by everyone under the tent, including the political leader, the pole. The canvas represents large-group identity.

Anna Freud (1954), in discussing the "widening scope of psychoanalysis," illustrated bias toward treating only neurotic patients instead of struggling with new technical problems. Her attitude could not be maintained. As time went on, with the influence of new theories, new psychoanalytic "schools," and other factors including economic ones, many psychoanalysts continued or began in greater numbers to treat individuals with narcissistic and borderline personality organizations, as well as individuals with extremely traumatic early childhood histories. This, and further realization that a child's mind does not evolve without his or her interactions with the mother and/or a mothering person, increased psychoanalysts' attention to pre-oedipal issues.

Some authors postulated that people experience their large group as a maternal ego ideal or a breast-mother who repairs narcissistic injuries (Anzieu, 1984; Chasseguet-Smirgel, 1973; Kernberg, 2003a, 2003b). It is possible that in individual psychology, the canvas of the tent can be perceived as a breast-mother and the pole can remain as a symbol of a primal father. But work in large-group psychology steered us toward a focus on the canvas of the tent representing the large-group identity that develops in childhood or adulthood and is shared by thousands or millions of people, including the political leader, the pole.

There are subgroups and subgroup identities, such as professional identities, or being followers of a sports team, under a typical large-group tent. A person can change a subgroup identity either with or without anxiety. After going through the adolescence passage, however, a person cannot change a core large-group identity that developed in childhood, even if he or she, due to special life experiences, wishes to hide or deny it (V. D. Volkan, 2018, 2020). If the person becomes an immigrant or refugee, his or her personal issues, along with the situation in the new country he or she comes to live in, may impact whether he or she adapts well and develops biculturalism. Some adults put themselves under a new tent when they become members of religious cults or terrorist organizations, and they modify the influence of their large-group identity that had developed in childhood.

A child is, to use Erik Erikson's (1966) term, a *generalist* as far as nationality, ethnicity, religion, or political ideology are concerned. Now let us look how a child stops being a "generalist" and develops a core large-group identity. Many scientific studies of recent decades illustrate that there is a psychobiological potential of "we-ness" and bias toward one's own kind (for example, see: Bloom, 2010; Emde, 1991; Purhonen et al., 2005; Stern, 1985).

Long ago, Sigmund Freud (1940a) noted that parents represent the greater society to their children. Children assimilate their core large-group identities and prejudices against the *other* by identifying with parents and other important people in their environments. Furthermore, parents and other important people "deposit" images of past historical events, heroes, and martyrs into their children's minds. When thousands or millions of children become receivers of the same or a similar deposited item, they begin to share "psychological DNA" linked to large-group identity.

As their minds develop, children slowly learn that certain things, such as the design and colors of their large group's flag, belong to their large group, and certain other things do not belong to their large group, such as the design and colors of the other's flag. After age two, children begin mending their "good" (libidinally invested) and "bad" (aggressively invested) images of important objects and corresponding self-images (Kernberg, 1976; V. D. Volkan, 1976) and become able to tolerate ambivalence. However, such integrations are not totally complete. Some self- and object images remain unintegrated, and the child finds ways to deal with these unintegrated images to avoid facing and feeling object relations tension. One psychological method a child uses to deal with this problem is to externalize his or her unintegrated self- and object images onto other persons or animate or inanimate objects.

Suitable targets of externalization

The people in the child's environment also help the child to find "permanent" reservoirs in which to keep the externalized unintegrated self- and object images. Such images, in the psychoanalytic literature, are known as *"bad"* (aggressively loaded) and *"good"* (libidinally loaded) unintegrated images. Since externalizations into such reservoirs are approved by the individuals important to the child, what is externalized will not boomerang, that is, will not be re-internalized by the child. These reservoirs are the *suitable targets of externalization* (V. D. Volkan, 1988). Libidinally loaded unmended objects and self-images are invested in one's own large-group symbols, while aggressively loaded unmended objects and self-images are externalized onto shared symbols of the other.

Once the child utilizes suitable targets of externalization, he or she slowly ceases to be a generalist. Here are two examples.

Case example of externalization 1

In the Mediterranean island of Cyprus, Cypriot Greeks and Cypriot Turks lived side by side for centuries until the island was *de facto* divided into two political entities in 1974. Greeks often raise pigs. Turkish children, like Greek children, invariably are drawn to farm animals, but imagine a Turkish child wanting to touch and love a piglet. His mother or other important individuals in the Turkish child's environment would strongly discourage him from playing with the piglet. For Moslem Turks, the pig is "dirty." The pig, as a cultural amplifier for the Greeks, does not belong to their large group. Now, the Turkish child finds a suitable target of externalization for his unwanted, aggressively contaminated, and unintegrated "*bad*" self- and object images. Since Moslem Turks do not eat pork, in a concrete sense, what is externalized into the image of the pig will not be re-internalized.

When the child unconsciously finds a suitable target for unintegrated "bad" self- and object images, the precursor of the other becomes established in the child's mind at an experimental level. The Turkish child at this point does not know what Greekness means. Sophisticated thoughts, perceptions, and emotions, and images of history about the other evolve much later without the individual's awareness that the first symbol of the other was in the service of helping him or her avoid feeling object relations tension. Since almost every Turkish child in Cyprus will use the same target, they will share the same precursor of the other.

Case example of externalization 2

Children also are given suitable targets as reservoirs for their "good" unintegrated self- and object relations. For example, a Finnish child uses the sauna as such a reservoir. Only when Finnish children grow up will they have sophisticated thoughts and feelings about Finnishness.

It is interesting that when there is an international conflict or a war-like situation, members of a large group who feel victimized regress and become involved in the creation of an *adult version* of suitable targets of externalization. For example, when Gaza fell under Israeli occupation, Palestinians began to carry small stones painted with the Palestinian flag's colors in their pockets. When facing humiliating external situations, they would reach in their pockets and touch the stones. Possessing these stones created a network of "we-ness", supported the large-group identity of Palestinians living in Gaza at that time, and separated their large-group identity from the Israelis' large-group identity.

We have already mentioned Peter Blos's (1979) description of "second individuation." During the adolescence passage period, an individual's large-group identity that evolved during childhood also becomes a core identity (V. D. Volkan, 1988, 1997, 2020). If a person migrates to another country after the adolescence passage, he or she must develop biculturalism to adapt to a new environment. Depending on the location where the child grows up, this large-group identity's focus will be on ethnicity, nationality, religion, or political ideology.

Large-group identity that develops in adulthood

New large-group identity also manifests when individuals are adults. Following a baseball team, working for a huge business organization, or belonging to the same academic profession does not force people to modify their core large-group identity developed in childhood.

In contrast, for members of religious cults or terrorist organizations, the investment in their core large-group identities that had developed in childhood drastically changes. These individuals exaggerate selected aspects of their childhood large-group identities by holding on to a restricted and special religious, nationalistic, or ideological belief. Sometimes they become believers of ideas that were not available in their childhood environments. In short, they give up sharing overall sentiments with people who had the same core childhood large-group identity but who have not made their specific new selections. Belonging to this second type of large-group identity in adulthood, members of religious cults or terrorist organizations lose their superego-imposed restrictions that are linked to the large-group identity that they acquired as children. They may take part in mass suicides or mass killings. A good example can be found in Vamık Volkan's book *Bloodlines: From Ethnic Pride to Ethnic Terrorism* (1997), where he describes Palestinian orphans who have underdeveloped personal identities and overdeveloped large-group identities:

> I had occasion to observe five children, all very young, who tended to stay together while playing in the courtyard. They had been rescued as infants from the massacres of some two

thousand unarmed Palestinian and Lebanese civilians by Israeli-backed phalange Christian militiamen at Sabra and Shatila, refugee camps in West Beirut ... Apparently their parents, before they were killed, had hidden the children to save them from being murdered. The children's real identities were unknown. They seemed "normal" when together, but when they were separated for the interview—through an interpreter—each one became agitated and experienced extreme difficulty relating to me and the others. One hallucinated acutely, and another began destroying the furniture. It was evident to me that these children did not have well-established individual identities. Being with others from Sabra and Shatila enabled them to appear normal ... ethnic identity dominated personal identity. The maintenance and protection of the group identity were psychological necessities. Many ... children and youths wanted to be military pilots so they could fly to the land of their ancestors and bomb enemy positions. ... While studying, playing, eating, watching television, and almost constantly hugging and kissing one another, the orphans gave the initial impression of being in a nonstop love fest. The children were healthy as long as they were Palestinian orphans, patching up one another's personality deficits. (pp. 149–150)

Large-group identity issues in the clinical setting

Large-group identity issues appear in the clinical setting not only when we deal with patients who are new immigrants. A young lady, Elisa, sought out psychoanalytic treatment. Soon after she was born, her Jewish parents moved to a conservative location in Virginia due to a job opportunity for the patient's father. At this location, there were not many Jewish residents, and the few Jewish individuals who did reside there were considered to be not as good as Christians. Elisa's parents decided to hide their religious large-group identity. They were "Jewish" only when they were in their home and without visitors. Later, they would teach their daughter to hide her Jewish identity. Their daughter grew up with this family "secret," graduated from a university, and married a Christian man. Hiding her Jewish identity from her husband became a disturbing issue for her, and she sought psychoanalytic treatment. As Elisa's treatment progressed, she told her husband how she had lied to him, went through a divorce, and established herself as a secure Jewish-American person successful in her own profession.

There are also stories of white patients from rich families living in the American South who, as small children, had two "mothers": the biological mother and the black nanny (V. D. Volkan, 2010, 2021a V. D. Volkan & Fowler, 2009). Later in life, these patients had trouble integrating "white" and "black" mother images, leading to psychological problems.

Harold Blum (1985) tells the story of a Jewish patient who came to him for re-analysis. This patient illustrated the extent to which mutual resistances may prevail when both the analyst and the analysand belong to the same large group that has been massively traumatized by an external historical event. Blum's patient's first analyst, who was Jewish, failed to "hear" their large group's trauma at the hand of the Nazis in his analysand's material. As a consequence, mutually sanctioned silence and denial pervaded the entire psychoanalytic experience, leaving unanalyzed residues of the Holocaust-related issues in the analysand's symptoms. At the present time, silence and denial related to the Holocaust during psychoanalytic clinical settings have disappeared due to intensive work on this subject by psychoanalysts such as Ilany Kogan (1995) and Ira Brenner (2019). (Also see: V. D. Volkan & Ast, 2001.)

CHAPTER 12

Traumas and transgenerational transmissions

In this chapter, we will focus on how traumas and other life events during childhood, as well as later periods of life, become connected by playing a role in an individual's developing various types of pathological symptoms. We will also focus on finding creative solutions.

Facing traumas during the developmental years

We can divide traumas that a person may face during his or her developmental years into six categories.

1. Traumas related to physical bodily deformities or mental disabilities with which a baby is born. Birth defects range from having a clubfoot or cleft lip to having spina bifida or Down syndrome. Genetic and epigenetic abnormalities, as well as structural and chemical pathologies of the body, including the brain, can be included here.
2. Traumas related to the child-mother (or mothering persons) interactions, such as those that take place when a mother suffers from postpartum depression and is unable to respond to a baby's emotional and physical needs.

3. Traumas occurring in the child's home, such as when he or she becomes a target for the angry outbursts of a parent or older sibling, his or her mother or other family member dies, or he or she is physically assaulted or sexually molested by a family member.

4. Traumas faced outside the child's home, such as by being humiliated in front of classmates by a teacher, physically assaulted or sexually abused by an adult, or involved in a car accident.

5. Traumas experienced due to drastic natural, social, or political events, such as facing huge devastation after an earthquake, belonging to an ethnic or racial large group that is oppressed, or becoming a refugee. Unfortunately, as we are writing this book, this type of trauma has become all too common. We are witnessing external trauma due to the Covid-19 pandemic and the invasion of Ukraine on the world stage, while those of us in the United States and other countries are experiencing political and social upheaval.

6. Traumas arising from images related to the suffering of previous generations along with the difficulty of dealing with such images (transgenerational transmissions).

Later, we will illustrate how traumas play a role in inducing unconscious and sometimes conscious fantasies in a child's mind.

Depositing and transgenerational transmissions

Anna Freud and Dorothy Burlingham's (1942) observation that children sensed their caregivers' anxiety during the German Luftwaffe bombings of London in World War II was mentioned above. Later observations on transferring anxiety from an adult to a child have found their way into theoretical formations. For example, in his work with severely regressed patients with schizophrenia, Harry Stack Sullivan (1962) theorized that this mental condition was caused primarily by the anxiety conveyed to these patients by their mothers in their early developmental years, though we now know that the genesis of schizophrenia is more complicated (K. Volkan & V. D. Volkan, 2022).

It is not only anxiety that travels from the mother or other primary caretaker to a developing child through the permeable boundary. Other psychological images and messages, such as a mother's unconscious fantasy, can also be deposited into her child.

"Depositing" is closely related to *identification* in childhood. In fact, it may even be called a variation of identification. But it is significantly different than identification proper. In identification, the child is the primary active partner in taking in and assimilating object images and related ego and superego functions from another person. In depositing, the other, an adult person, more actively pushes his or her specific self- and internalized object images and related ego and superego functions into the developing self-representation of the child. In other words, the other uses the child, mostly unconsciously, as a reservoir for certain self- and object images and ego and superego tasks that belong to that adult. The experiences that created these mental images in the adult are not "accessible" to the child, but instead are deposited or pushed into the child without the experiential/contextual framework from which they originally arose (V. D. Volkan, 1987; V. D. Volkan & Ast, 1997; V. D. Volkan et Al., 2002).

One area where the concept of depositing can be illustrated clearly is the so-called *replacement child* phenomenon (Ainslie & Solyom, 1986; Budak, 2015; Cain & Cain, 1964; Green & Solnit, 1964; Legg & Sherick, 1976; Poznanski, 1972; V. D. Volkan & Ast, 1997). A mother (or mothering person) has an internalized formed image of her child (or another relative) who has died. She deposits or transgenerationally transports (Kestenberg & Brenner, 1996; Kogan, 1995; Laub & Auerhahn, 1993) this image into the developing self-representation of her next-born child, usually born after the first child's death. The second child, the replacement child, has no actual experience with or image of the dead sibling. The mother, who has an image of the dead child, treats the second one as the reservoir where the dead child can be kept "alive." Accordingly, the mother (mostly unconsciously) encourages the second child to develop ego tasks to protect and main-tain what has been pushed into him or her. The second child may or may not succeed in doing so.

If the task is successful, the replacement child will not exhibit psychopathology. Sometimes the assimilated idealized deposited representation may become a motivation for the individual to excel in certain areas of life experiences. If this task is not successful, replacement children may develop an unintegrated self-representation and therefore a borderline, narcissistic, or even psychotic personality organization (V. D. Volkan, 1987; K. Volkan & V. D. Volkan, 2022).

The mother or other caretaker who deposits the mental image of a dead child (or other dead relatives) into the developing self of a child is herself or himself suffering from difficulty of mourning and is thus traumatized. In the replacement child phenomenon, there may also be some depositing of the depositor's injured self-image into the child's self. Some adults may actively, but mostly unconsciously, push their own traumatized self- and traumatized object images, whether they are connected to a concrete loss or not, into developing self-representations of their children. Although the child who becomes a reservoir is not a completely passive partner, it is the other (the adult) who initiates this transfer of images. There are many historical examples of replacement children, including Elvis Presley and Adolf Hitler, who developed narcissistic or borderline personality organization (Bromberg, 1971; K. Volkan, 1994b, 2021a; V. D. Volkan, 2006a).

Rescue fantasies and replacement child phenomenon

In psychoanalytic clinical practice, we observe "rescue fantasies" in patients whose families had traumatic losses. During their childhood, and/or while going through the adolescence passage, such patients had mothers (or other caretakers with mothering functions) who were depressed, missing, or otherwise unable to provide good-enough mothering. At the same time, these children or youngsters could not "reach up" to a father or father figure to find a nurturing object. Their unconscious fantasy of saving the mother from her depression and bringing her back to function as a mother is to induce an illusion of having a good mothering experience. The "mental content" of a rescue fantasy may lead to maladaptive or adaptive compromise formations during the individual's adulthood (Abend, 2008; Arlow, 1969; Beres, 1962; Inderbitzin & Levy, 1990; V. D. Volkan, 1981, 2010).

As we stated above, in the replacement child phenomenon, there may also be some depositing of the depositor's injured self-image into the child's self. Some adults may actively, but mostly unconsciously, push their own traumatized self- and traumatized object images, whether they relate to a concrete loss or not, into developing self-representations of their children. The actual memories of the trauma belong to these adults; their children have no experience with the trauma. Clearly, memories belonging to one person cannot be transmitted to another person, but an adult can deposit traumatized self- and object images as well as others, such as realistic or imagined object images that are formed in the depositor's mind as a response to trauma, into a child's self-representation. This process may or may not be a source of pathology depending on how the child handles what had been "deposited" by the traumatized adult into his or her internal world.

George Pollock (1975) gathered data on artists, scientists, and political leaders and pundits concerning their childhood experiences with death. He found that loss does not necessarily account for the creative act or the creative product, but the creative act may be given direction by childhood loss. Similar findings appeared in other psychoanalytic studies (Hamilton, 1969, 1979; Plank & Plank, 1978; Wolfenstein, 1973). Vamık Volkan (2010) concluded, as George Pollock had done, that rescue fantasies have pushed many individuals to search out leadership roles, including political ones.

What we need to keep in mind is that some leaders influenced by such a fantasy become *reparative* leaders who increase the self-esteem of their ethnic, national, religious, or ideological large groups without hurting and destroying or oppressing another large group. Kemal Atatürk was a replacement child; his mother lost three children and her husband when her son was a child. Vamık Volkan and Norman Itzkowitz (1984) describe in detail how the Turkish leader verbalized his rescue fantasy in words and deeds. He became the "savior" of the Turks after the collapse of the Ottoman Empire.

Other political leaders become *destructive* leaders who deliberately initiate inhumane actions and oppress and injure innocent people, primarily to satisfy their own and their followers' narcissism (V. D. Volkan, 2004, 2020). Vamık Volkan and Jana Javakhishvili (2022) described Vladimir Putin as a replacement child and illustrated how the Russian leader, in his open statements and actions, has linked Russia—as well as the image of the Soviet Union—to the time and place where his family lived. There, surrounded by the Nazis, he experienced many losses and became preoccupied with burials and graveyards. He evolved as a destructive leader.

Anne Ancelin Schützenberger's "ancestor syndrome" (1998), Judith Kestenberg's term "transgenerational transposition" (1982), and Haydée Faimberg's description of "the telescoping of generations" (2005) all refer to "depositing" traumatized images. By performing the act of "depositing," the depositors externalize their troublesome images into another person in order to become "free" of the troublesome images carried within them. In other instances, depositors externalize the wished-for images to keep themselves "alive" in someone in the next generation. Through "depositing," the adult attempts to free themselves from the mental conflicts and anxiety associated with deposited images. On the other hand, the children, who are a reservoir, are given (metapsychologically speaking) a *psychological gene* that influences their self-representation, and thus their sense of identity. This psychological gene may or may not be a source of pathology depending on how the child handles what the traumatized adult "deposited" into the child's internal world.

CHAPTER 13

Two case stories illustrating transgenerational transmissions

In this chapter we tell Vamık Volkan's story of a replacement child that was one of his cases. The full story of her treatment appears in his book *Linking Objects and Linking Phenomena* (1981). Then we will illustrate depositing (transgenerational transmission) with another case that Volkan supervised.

A replacement child

Frances was a college student in her mid-twenties when she became a psychoanalytic patient. She spoke of having become aware four years earlier of presences around her, especially when she was alone in her own room. At first, what she called "the spirits" did not speak, but one night, when a candle in her room "lit itself" she felt suffused with warmth at what she interpreted as a signal that her spectral visitors were good spirits. She was told by the spirits that they had come to make her feel better. Then they took command of her life, counseling her when to smile, when to blow her nose, when to take a vacation, etc. However, Frances was able to continue to attend her classes at the college while having no close friends.

Frances was an adopted and only child. Her adoptive mother had miscarried after a five-month pregnancy, and her physician, aware of her strong desire for a child, had later arranged for her to take Frances home from the hospital as a four-day-old infant. The adoptive mother had had a hysterectomy after her miscarriage; her health had not been good, and there were indications that she had been depressed for months after miscarrying. The maternal grandmother had taken over the mothering of the adopted infant during her first months of life; the maternal grandparents had lived near Frances's adoptive parents at that time. When the grandfather died, Frances was eight, and the grandmother began living in the home of her daughter. As a child, Frances had been given no information about her biological parents. When she started her psychoanalytic treatment, her grandmother was an invalid who still lived in her daughter's house.

A few months after starting psychoanalytic treatment Frances revealed that when she was five, she amused herself by making a stage with wooden blocks and having toy singers perform on it. "Of course, the blocks belonged to *him*," she explained. This "him" turned out to be her mother's younger and only brother, a pilot shot down in Europe during World War II. When she told me his name, I realized that *Frances* had been given its feminine version. Her dead uncle's name was *Francis*.

Francis had been "God's gift to the world," according to Frances's grandmother. Her grandmother would tell my patient, "God took him away and then He gave us you." The old lady even referred to my patient as "a reincarnation of Francis." My patient felt that spirits lived on an astral plane, on the highest level of which lived Francis. I began to realize that my patient's preoccupation with spirits, astral planes, and reincarnation had something to do with her being chosen as a "replacement child" by her parents, and especially by her grandmother.

After some time passed, I learned that Francis, along with the plane's two other occupants, had been burned beyond recognition in the fiery crash. When the bodies had been sent home, it was impossible to identify which was the body of Francis. At the funeral of the three men, the grandmother, "feeling the hand of God on her shoulder," had been able to see the ascent of her son's image from one of the coffins. She had stopped crying; struck by the recognition of her son's ghostly body and the realization that he was both dead and alive.

Although Frances had initially been chosen to replace a dead fetus, she was also the replacement for the dead pilot who would have been replaced by the child lost in miscarriage. Talk about the dead pilot was never-ending in Frances's home, whereas there was no mention of the aborted infant. Frances associated the "immortal" representation of the dead chiefly with her perception of the dead pilot.

It was soon after the shocking death of the pilot Francis that my patient's adoptive mother married her husband, also a pilot. Interestingly, my patient herself became a pilot, learning to fly when she was sixteen. After the grandfather's death and the grandmother's move into her daughter's house, the house became a monument to the dead pilot, whose picture hung on almost every wall.

Frances was chosen by both her grandmother and mother to replace Francis, and their perception of this substitute as half-alive and half-dead, half-girl and half-boy, passed into the child's self-concept as she developed through interactions with the mothering persons, making integration of a total self-concept and corresponding internalized object images impossible.

Frances was fascinated with Edgar Allan Poe (1809–1849), the death-obsessed American writer and poet known to have faced early childhood loss with the death of his mother. My patient recalled Poe's short story, *The Masque of the Red Death*, which was first published in 1842. This story tells of a prince and his followers hiding away in a castle to escape a pestilence. In the story, the pestilence overtakes the characters despite their precautions, resulting in blood springing from the pores of their faces.

Frances spent inordinate periods of time gazing at her face on the mirror. She said that spirits made her unable to see pimples on her face. But she knew that she had pimples. She spoke of frantic masturbation when as a girl she heard that sexual activity keeps the face from breaking out, but she reported that her face had been disfigured despite her efforts. Frances recalled having a dream about Edgar Allan Poe's story. In the dream she was in a castle, afflicted by the Red Death, a terrible plague, but with its characteristic disfigurement in only half of her face. (It should be noted that Frances was my patient decades ago, well before the Covid-19 pandemic.)

It seemed as though Frances was wondering if her face, or half of her face, was, or would be like the dead pilot's face. During her sessions, it was helpful to have her stay focused on the pilot's story. It was at this time that Frances revealed how all the plane's three occupants had been burned beyond recognition.

The next day in her session Frances cried out, "My heart is beating!" To which it was confirmed, "You are alive!" It was worth trying to see how much connection Frances made between her symptoms (talking to spirits; being half in this world and half on an astral plane; being half-girl and half-boy; half-deformed, half-not-deformed). Although the attempt was made cautiously, it was premature. Frances let it be known that she was not ready to hear such things. "If I don't believe in spirits there is something wrong with my chemistry," she said. "And if something is wrong with my chemistry that is unchangeable." This led to the realization of how Frances was perceived as a replacement child.

The working alliance with Frances bloomed, and she expressed how much she appreciated helping her make sense of the bizarre and disorganized material she had brought to her treatment. A warmth and aliveness in her became noticeable. Fortified by the therapeutic alliance, Frances talked about the movie *Night of the Living Dead* (Romero, 1968). This popular horror movie is about seven people who are trapped in a farmhouse and are assaulted by cannibalistic, undead ghouls. As a teenager Frances was fascinated by this movie. "It was like a Frankenstein or Dracula entertainment, in which the dead ate the living in order to live themselves," she said. It was reflected to her that Francis ate her to stay alive, and she ate him in turn to identify with him. She said that when she felt a spirit enter her for the first time it felt as though cancer were eating her inside.

The next day Frances missed an hour for the first time. Two days later she said how badly she felt over failing to appear but explained that she had had "a sore throat." This was interpreted as her incorporative anxieties, cannibalistic fantasies, and her defensive refusal to eat meat. During this hour, she felt extreme anxiety, and as the hour concluded, she let herself identify with the dead by feeling her body turn cold. Once the experience was over, she burst out sobbing. She had passed the test—having done something under the gaze of her observing ego that formerly she had done unconsciously, with accompanying pathological defenses and adaptations. This occurred at the end of her first year of her treatment.

A legacy of the 1942 Bataan Death march

Gregory was an American sailor during WWII who worked on a submarine where he oversaw the submarine's torpedoes. The Japanese captured him when he was stationed in the Philippines, and he participated in the Bataan Death March in the spring of 1942. The American and Filipino prisoners were forced to march sixty-five miles in the boiling sun while Japanese soldiers beat them with whips and rifle butts. Thousands died. After that, Gregory was in a Japanese prison camp where he witnessed and experienced unbelievable cruelty until the end of the war. He observed the beheadings of fellow prisoners by swords; he buried his dead friends in shallow graves and reburied them when floods brought their corpses to the surface of the earth.

Soon after he returned to the United States a thin and haggard figure, Gregory became friendly with a woman whose husband had left her when their only child, Peter, was three weeks old. Gregory moved in with her, the woman's mother, and Peter, who then was under the age of two, traumatized, overfed, and obese.

During Peter's early childhood, Gregory stayed at home while the women went to work, thereby assuming the major parenting role for Peter. A few years later, Gregory married Peter's mother and adopted Peter as his son. The newlyweds moved to a new house, leaving behind the boy's grandmother, who died before Peter reached puberty. Gregory rarely spoke of his horrific experiences during the war and continued to be his stepson's primary caregiver during the boy's developmental years.

Depositing and externalization were Gregory's main defense mechanisms that made it possible for him live a "normal" life in the United States following the unspeakable traumas he had experienced overseas during the war. After he and his family moved to their new house, Gregory built a multi-storied purple martin birdhouse in the garden. For decades this birdhouse remained as a permanent fixture there. Gregory took infinite pains to paint (and repaint when the old paint faded) numbers on each of the many "apartments" the bird families occupied. Every year it was full of birds. When their eggs hatched, the birds fed their fledglings and helped them fly to freedom when they were ready.

Yearly, Gregory put a band on one leg of every baby bird after it was hatched. Each band was numbered to correspond with the number on its family's "apartment" in the birdhouse. If a baby bird had an untimely fall from the birdhouse, Gregory would know to which "apartment" it belonged and would then return the baby bird to its proper nest. This was extremely important, because if a baby bird was rescued by a human, but returned to the wrong nest, it would be rejected by the adult birds in that "apartment" and would certainly die.

The purple martin birdhouse symbolically represented Gregory's Japanese prison camp where he suffered a great deal and was exposed to the deaths of his comrades almost daily. Gregory saw to it that no baby birds would die while occupying his birdhouse. He changed "the function" of the image of his prison camp; he had created a "camp" where occupants, the baby birds that were reservoirs of Gregory's and his comrades' helpless images, were not allowed to die.

When Peter, Gregory's stepson, was in his mid-forties, he sought psychoanalytic treatment with a male psychoanalyst of Peter's age for a sadistic narcissistic personality organization and bulimia. Only after Peter had been on the psychoanalyst's couch for a while was the stepfather's story revealed. When Peter started his psychoanalysis, Gregory was in his seventies and still seemed to have a "normal" life (V. D. Volkan, 2014).

During his psychoanalysis, Peter realized that his stepfather treated him like he treated his baby birds, and he described how Gregory had been preoccupied with making little Peter strong. To accomplish this, Gregory prescribed certain tasks for him and taught him how to exercise, lose weight, and develop an athletic body. When Peter was in his early teens, Gregory introduced him to guns and taught him how to hunt. Soon, using his contacts, he made sure that Peter enrolled in a military school. After graduation as a military man, Peter served in the war in Vietnam. Later, as a civilian, he worked for the military defense industry and became rich. Although adult Peter's hobby was hunting, he was *not* a sportsman. Whenever he felt anxious, he would kill many animals. Since he had a great deal of money, he could afford to hire a helicopter for his hunting trips, and on many occasions, he would heartlessly shoot at a herd of deer from above.

Peter and his psychoanalyst slowly began to understand that Gregory had deposited his "hunted" self-image (injured, humiliated, and rendered helpless in the war) into the little boy's developing self-representation.

Indeed, there was a nice "fit" between Gregory's deposited injured image and little Peter's own obese helpless image in a home dominated by intrusive women. When Gregory gave tasks to his stepson—indeed acting like his "trainer," he made him (in fact he deposited his own image into little Peter as well) a "hunter" instead of the "hunted" one, reversing his helplessness and making the boy feel omnipotently powerful.

Peter's understanding of his identification with Gregory and his role as a "reservoir" for his stepfather's injured image became clear when he and his psychoanalyst examined the various meanings of one of Peter's major preoccupations as an adult. Gregory had been preoccupied with his birdhouse and its occupants, and adult Peter became preoccupied with a special room in his house and its occupants. Peter had built a huge room with trophies of his hunts hung on the walls. By the creation of such a room, he unconsciously repeated the "memories" of the prisoner Gregory surrounded by his dead comrades. His hobby also included one of the tasks Gregory had given to him—to resurrect the dead and change the function of the prison camp as Gregory had done when he protected the lives of baby birds. Thus, Peter took pains to make his trophies look "alive" through skillful taxidermy, spending considerable time and money on taxidermists to achieve this illusion.

Throughout his treatment, Peter had a repeating dream in which he saw himself walking on water like Jesus Christ. Only toward the termination phase of his treatment did he have a new version of this repeating dream. In the dream, he was not walking on water but on a submarine that was lying a few inches below the surface of the water. Peter realized that the submarine stood for Gregory, who had worked on a submarine just before the Japanese captured him. This new version of his repeating dream gave Peter the firm insight that Gregory had supported his omnipotent self-image. In fact, he was an extension of Gregory and was the old man's "reservoir." Peter was in the last phase of his treatment when he had yet another version of his repeating dream. In this one, the submarine dived, Peter fell in the water, and he had to swim to shore as an "average" individual. Changes in Peter's repeating dreams inform us about the story of an individual psychological life and his or her wished for as well as actual changes in his or her internal world.

CHAPTER 14

Dreams and unconscious fantasies

Sigmund Freud (1900a, 1918b, 1933a) described dreams as another kind of remembering. According to Freud, dreams have two parts—the manifest and the latent. The manifest aspect of the dream is what you remember when you wake up. The latent aspect is the true meaning of the dream—forbidden fantasies, wishes fulfilled, secret desires, etc. All of these appear in the manifest aspects of the dream in disguised or distorted form and are usually unrecognizable as the latent aspects. The disguising and distorting of the latent aspects of a dream occur in four ways through:

Condensation—two or more latent aspects are combined into one manifest aspect.

Displacement—emotion or desire for a latent aspect in a dream is displaced onto an unrelated or meaningless manifest aspect.

Symbolism—the manifest aspects use symbols to make the more overtly sexual latent aspects more acceptable to consciousness as manifest aspects of a dream (e.g., key in the lock).

Secondary revision—where we revise the dream in its manifest state to make it more logical. Contradictions are covered up, absurdities explained.

Freud believed that all dreams represent unfulfilled wishes in their latent form. His main technique to work back from the manifest content of the dream to the latent content was "free association." The patient would lie on a couch facing away from the analyst and recall whatever manifest aspects of the dream came to mind. In a hypnagogic state, and with the analyst's help via interpretation, the manifest aspects of the dream could be unraveled and the latent content—that is, the true meaning of the dream and its "wish"—would be revealed.

As we have already mentioned, Freud described what is known in the literature as "day residue." Impressions derived from the real world, even insignificant ones—such as seeing a police cruiser chasing a speeding car on the highway, or passing a billboard depicting a smiling woman holding a milk bottle—join infantile aggressive or sexual wishes to initiate the content of dreams. Also, what is discussed during a therapy session can function as day residue.

There are common dream symbols, such as a snake stands for a penis and a cave for a mother's womb. A psychoanalytic clinician cannot fully understand each dream the patient reports. However, listening to dreams is important for psychoanalytic clinicians. For example, noticing the changes of Peter's repeating dreams clearly illustrated the changes in Peter's internal world. We will refer to more dreams—as well as daydreams—in the stories of other patients and illustrate how paying attention to them enriches the way in which psychoanalytic treatment is conducted.

Some cases (like Peter's) illustrate how dreams may tell us about the state of a patient's mind. Coming to treatment and some therapy sessions play the role of day residue. Sometimes a patient's "first dream" makes a summary of the patient's mental conflicts that will be dealt with in therapy. Sometimes dreams illustrate patients' transferences and attempts to resolve a conflict or resistances.

Unconscious fantasies

Sigmund Freud (1908a) described two types of unconscious fantasies: "Unconscious phantasies have been unconscious all along and have been formed in the unconscious; or—as is more often the case—they were once conscious phantasies, daydreams, and have been purposely forgotten and have become unconscious through 'repression'" (p. 161).

Melanie Klein and her followers emphasized Freud's first kind of unconscious fantasy and maintained that unconscious "phantasies" are inherited. Technically the term *phantasy* is used by Kleinians to refer to the state of an infant's mind. Phantasies are nonverbal, largely unconscious, and derived from the drives. They begin as psychic representations of instinctual drives and may subsequently become elaborated into well-formed wishes or defenses against internal dangers and anxiety throughout childhood and into adulthood (Klein, 1932, 1946; Segal, 1973). The word *fantasy*, on the other hand, is used to denote daydreams, reveries, wishes, or needs and can be conscious or unconscious. Not everyone in psychoanalytic circles makes a distinction between these two words. Kleinians say that since instinctual drives are present at birth, some crude phantasy such as creating a "bad breast" exists at the beginning of life.

Hanna Segal (1973) states:

> The first hunger and the instinctual striving to satisfy that hunger are accompanied by the phantasy of an object capable of satisfying that hunger. As phantasies derive directly from instincts on the borderline between the somatic and psychical activity, these original phantasies are experienced as somatic as well as mental phenomena. (p. 13).

It is difficult to imagine a newborn baby's mind evolving a phantasy that can later be put into words. By using words, psychoanalysts describe the experiences of a newborn baby as they understand them.

A child's ability to develop an "understanding" of a traumatic event or a series of traumatic events depends on the phase-specific ego functions available to the child and on his or her relations with important others involved in the traumatic event. When a child is in the very early stages, he or she contaminates this "understanding" with primary process thinking. This "understanding," initiated by an external event or series of events, is a collection of cognitions, affects, danger signals, wish fulfillment, and primitive defenses against wishes that are influenced by whichever psychological developmental tasks the child is dealing with at the time. These "phantasies" (if an early stage) or "fantasies" linked to trauma or traumas do not refer to a formed logical thought process. As the child grows, he or she starts forming a thought process linked to experiencing a traumatic event or a repeating traumatic experience. The thought content, unformed or formed, usually is later repressed. But when they are adults, individuals may respond to the theme of the unconscious phantasy or fantasy. During psychoanalytic treatment, the adult patient and the therapist bring the storyline of an unconscious phantasy or fantasy to consciousness. Because phantasies may evolve into fantasies, it becomes difficult to make fine distinctions between them. For this reason, we will use the term *fantasy* as the umbrella term for both phantasy and fantasy.

Psychoanalysts and psychoanalytically oriented psychotherapists observe conscious and unconscious fantasies and their continuing influence on the adult individual's mind. These fantasies can be called oral, anal, phallic, or oedipal.

Oral-level unconscious/conscious fantasies relate to primary thought process-influenced relationships with "good" and "bad" breasts and acts of swallowing (for example, getting pregnant by swallowing) or biting (for example, fantasy about a *vagina dentata*, that is, a vagina with teeth).

Anal-level fantasies include references equating hostile emotions with bowel movements, delivering children through the anus, creating fecal penises, and emotional constipation.

At the phallic level, the child may have fantasies about inserting a sword, a symbol of a penis, into the rival's body. Castration fantasies are linked to the Oedipus complex. The so-called "family romance" fantasy (Freud, 1909c) usually takes place at the oedipal phase. The child imagines that he or she is the offspring of another couple, a noble or famous couple, from whom he or she was separated in infancy. The child wishes to join this fantasized couple.

Many unconscious fantasies cannot be easily "classified" by psychosexual developmental terminology and belong *only* to the individuals who have them. They occur especially if the initiation of the unconscious fantasy is due to a trauma or a collection of traumas specific to the child. The following case that was supervised by Vamık Volkan illustrates this.

Case example of unconscious fantasy

Maria was in her thirties and felt that she was having a comfortable life. One day she had a disagreement with another female coworker who was about two years younger than her. Maria shouted at the younger woman and expressed her aggression openly. A week later a stranger hit the younger coworker, by accident, with her car. The younger woman was taken to a hospital and was expected to die. However, she survived and later returned to work.

Eight months after the younger woman's accident, Maria sought psychoanalytic psychotherapy treatment. She told her psychotherapist that she suddenly and unexpectedly began suffering from depressive feelings. She was feeling guilty even for minor angry feelings caused by minor incidents. At the beginning of her psychotherapy there was no reference to her verbal argument with the coworker.

A year after her psychoanalytic psychotherapy started, Maria could describe the unconscious fantasy that had caused her unexpected psychological problems. When she was seven years old, she had measles. As she recovered, her only sibling, a sister who was two years younger, also contracted measles. The parents were not financially capable to hire help. They locked Maria, their seven-year-old daughter, in a room for many hours day after day while looking after Maria's sick younger sister. Being locked up in a room and having no one coming to comfort her when she was shouting and asking for "freedom" was very scary for Maria as a child. Her sister had complications and died. Maria was once more locked in a room while the parents went through funeral arrangements and the burial of their younger daughter. During the following years, the parents talked to others in front of Maria about how they blamed Maria for giving measles to her deceased younger sister.

Now the patient recalled how when she first met her coworker some years before they had had an open argument, and she had a thought: "If my sister did not die, she would look like this woman, whose eye color is identical to my dead sister's eye color." Maria and her psychotherapist now understood how hearing that her coworker may die stimulated her childhood unconscious fantasy that resulted in the development of her depressive symptoms. Now she and her psychotherapist could put words to the patient's unconscious fantasy: "I am a murderer; I can kill people."

Womb fantasies

Vamık Volkan and Gabriele Ast (1997) examined what can be named "womb fantasies." Unconscious womb fantasies usually appear in older children who experience their mother's pregnancy as traumatic and the birth of their younger siblings as an intrusion. When these older children, as adults, undergo psychoanalysis, they often describe previously unconscious womb fantasies connected with sibling rivalries; the storyline usually involves the child imagining entering his or her mother's belly and killing the fetus so that he or she will be the sole occupant of the womb. This causes a conflict: the wish to "kill" the fetus clashes with a fear of losing the mother and her love (because she is the carrier of the fetus) or of being punished by the superego. The conflict produces anxiety, and the child develops two mental mechanisms that occur simultaneously: displacement and avoidance. The child, or the adult who still has the unconscious fantasy, displaces the mother's womb onto an enclosed space, such as a closet, an airplane, or a cave, and then avoids being there. In other words, he or she develops symptoms of claustrophobia.

There are variations on this theme. Sometimes the patient projects his or her aggression onto the fetus and then is afraid to enter the mother's womb (enclosed space) even while wishing to do so, because on entering it, the patient will face a fetus made ferocious by his or her own projections.

Volkan and Ast described adults who had anxiety entering a cave that symbolizes the mother's womb. They also referred to other adult patients who, in a counterphobic way, developed a hobby exploring caves. The storyline of a typical womb fantasy is: "I want to be my mother's only child in her womb. I will enter there and kill my sibling, but my sibling in turn may kill me."

Rescue fantasies

Not all unconscious fantasies cause psychological problems for individuals when they become adults. The mental content of an unconscious fantasy, even if it is repressed, may lead to maladaptive or adaptive compromise formations (Abend, 1990; Arlow, 1969; Beres, 1962; Inderbitzin & Levy, 1990; V. D. Volkan & Javakhishvili, 2022). We can refer to these as "rescue fantasies" that may have a lifelong influence for creativity and may direct the adult individual to seek certain social/ professional roles such as leadership positions, including political leadership.

A child may develop a rescue fantasy, for example, when his or her mother is depressed or suffering from a physical illness or when he or she senses anxiety in the family due to financial or other external factors. In the fantasy, the child turns a depressed mother into a "good" mother or finds a way to raise the family's living conditions. Stanley Olinick (1980) wondered what makes a person pursue a career as a psychoanalyst. He wrote about how unconscious rescue fantasies play a key role in directing individuals to become psychoanalysts.

Actualization of an unconscious fantasy

Actualization of an unconscious fantasy (V. D. Volkan, 2004, 2010) occurs when the actual trauma is severe or a series of actual traumas are accumulated, and when they interfere with "the usual restriction of fantasy only or mostly to the psychological realm" (V. D. Volkan & Ast, 2001, p. 569). The individual continues to experience symbols or objects of displacement representing various aspects of the actualized fantasies as "protosymbols" (Werner & Kaplan, 1963). That is to say, to this individual, the symbols *are* in actuality what they represent. The following case, which was. ... Volkan, gives an example of these ideas.

Case example of actualization of an unconscious fantasy

Smith, living on the East Coast of the United States, started his psychoanalytic treatment for panic and depressive states when he was fifty years old. Smith had never been married and from adolescence was inhibited around women and men of authority. He was suffering from premature ejaculation and erectile dysfunction, except when he was with a woman named Mary who lived on the West Coast of the United States. Although they lived over 2000 miles apart, the two had been sexually involved for a few decades. He would have an urgent impulse to fly and visit Mary again and again, although such actions were expensive and interfered with Smith's routine work. He described his impulse to be with Mary not as a wish, but as a most "puzzling need." From aspects of Smith's life story, we will come to understand Smith's repeated visits to Mary as an actualization of his unconscious fantasy of being castrated.

Smith was the third of three sons born to his parents. His brothers were two and six years older respectively. He described his mother, an elementary school teacher, as a passive, waif-like woman who was utterly bereft of maternal qualities. She openly told him that she never loved his father and would have divorced him if it were not for him and his brothers. His father worked as a foreman in a shipyard until his religious conversion in his late forties prompted him to resign this job and open a Christian bookstore. Smith described his father as a self-important man who disdained his sons, especially the two younger ones. Whenever his knowledge, opinions, or decisions were questioned, the father would fly into a rage. Smith thought his father an arrogant fool, although in his presence he never gave the slightest hint that he nurtured such a sentiment because he was so afraid of him.

Eight-year-old Smith had placed his hand on a log being chopped by his fourteen-year-old brother when the tip of his finger was lopped off. The oldest brother also tried to sodomize Smith after he emerged from a shower several months later. Smith's oldest brother was sadistic. When the parents were not around, Smith's brother would taunt and tease him mercilessly. Sometimes these verbal assaults would turn physical and this older brother would savagely beat the hapless Smith.

Shortly after Smith's finger was cut off, his father noticed a swollen area near his son's groin. Smith was seen by a doctor, who diagnosed an inguinal hernia about two inches from his penis. He received a hernia repair and remained in the hospital for several days to recuperate from this surgical procedure. Around this same time, his teacher decided that she would have her male students come to school dressed in girls' clothes. This so terrified Smith that he went into "a tailspin of panic." He complained to the principal who canceled this ill-conceived stunt. Smith's finger being cut by his sadistic brother, his being abused by the same brother, his undergoing surgery, and his being asked to dress like a girl all actualized Smith's castration anxiety.

Returning to Smith's *need* to visit Mary that had continued after he entered psychoanalytic psychotherapy, Smith declared that he had no intention of marrying Mary, but he had to be with her, especially following an event that made him feel humiliated, such as a problem he faced in his business or his experience being treated badly by an older male waiter at a restaurant.

Smith was well into the first year of his psychoanalytic psychotherapy when he informed his psychotherapist, almost as an aside, how his trips to be with Mary were directly related to the actualization of his castration fantasy. Upon his return from a weekend trip to the West Coast, Smith opened his session by saying, "We [meaning him and Mary] feed off each other. But what we really have most in common is our deformed little finger." It was then that the psychotherapist learned that Mary too had part of her finger missing.

Smith described how he and Mary would put together their cut fingers, as if one cut finger was an extension of the other cut finger, before having sex. Then Smith would not have erectile dysfunction or premature ejaculation. It seemed that two half fingers make a whole finger (whole penis) and that Smith, through a mental fusion of the two fingers, was undoing his actualized castration. This was why he needed to fly to the West Coast again and again.

A child may also develop actualized—Maria Bergmann (1982) and Ilany Kogan (1995) use the term "concretized"—unconscious fantasies as a result of identifying with parents, other relatives, or the large group (i.e., ethnic group) with which he or she is associated, who have sustained massive traumatic experiences, such as surviving the Holocaust (I. Brenner, 2019; V. D. Volkan et al., 2002). If such a person enters psychoanalysis as an adult, and if the storyline of his or her fantasy becomes available to him or her, that individual will have difficulty differentiating where his or her (now conscious) fantasy ends and where reality begins. For this person, then, keeping the transference development limited to the psychological realm will be difficult. Such an individual's therapeutic regression will need to take him or her to the point at which the unconscious fantasy became "actualized." It is as if the patient must "go back" to the time at which the mental "content" and the external reality originally converged to reestablish the difference between what belongs to an unconscious fantasy and what belongs to the external world.

We must add here that a patient's hearing the content of the unconscious fantasy, especially if it is an actualized one, during treatment does
not quickly lead to an intrapsychic change in the patient. The content
may need to come alive in the transference development. Sometimes
patients become involved in "therapeutic plays" to work through their
problems, which is the topic of the following chapter.

CHAPTER 15

Therapeutic play

In this chapter we will illustrate a patient's involvement in an activity, a "therapeutic play," that is used to tame, modify, and master the influence of a mental conflict or an unconscious fantasy, especially an actualized one, after the mental conflict or fantasy was interpreted and no longer unconscious. Then the psychoanalytic clinician will interpret the meaning and the aim of the therapeutic play.

Patients themselves, not the psychoanalytic clinician, initiate a therapeutic play. In therapeutic play, specific activities continue for weeks or months. The patient's preoccupation with and reporting of these activities to the psychoanalytic clinician becomes the central focus of verbal communication from session to session. The therapeutic play comes to an end in a way that is a *new experience* for the patient internally. Vamık Volkan's account of one of his cases illustrates this.

Constructing a Viking ship

Klaus, who had a severe obsessional neurosis, was in his thirties when he started his psychoanalysis with me. He was born after his parents immigrated to the United States, and he was their only offspring. As a child, Klaus was left alone much of the time since his parents had to work in their store to earn some money.

As his analysis progressed, the initiation of Klaus's obsessional neurosis, which had occurred when he was at the pubertal age of twelve, became clear. At that time, the family moved to a new city, and for some months lived in an apartment so small that the whole family slept in the same room. One night, when the child lay in his bed that stood alongside his parents' bed, the father unexpectedly turned on the light, and the youngster caught a glimpse of his mother preparing for intercourse by putting Vaseline on her vagina. Although the light had been quickly extinguished, in psychoanalysis Klaus gradually recognized incestuous wishes and fears that were mobilized. He recalled that during the night after this traumatic incident he had lain in bed listening intently for any sound from his parents' bed. He also recalled measuring in his mind in an obsessional way the distance between his bed and his parents' bed.

The move to the new location did not work out for the family, and soon after this incident they returned to their original city. By then, Klaus had a severe obsessional neurosis, and one day, after hearing a schoolmate call another a "motherfucker," his symptoms were exacerbated in reference to his reawakened incestuous conflict. Things might have been all right for him except that his neurosis crystallized when he broke into a theater with some friends as a prank and a man surprised by their break-in had a fatal heart attack. Klaus blamed himself for this old man's death. Unconsciously, his wish to get rid of his father was actualized. Klaus's obsessional thoughts about being a murderer generalized to the point that when he read about a murder in the paper, he obsessionally thought of himself as the person who committed it.

His symptoms were in remission when he married in his twenties. He proceeded to find an older man, a partner, to take him under his wing. As long as he submitted himself to this father figure, he could not become a "motherfucker." When he learned that his wife was having an affair with his partner, he began to have angry outbursts. After stopping his partnership with the older man and getting a divorce from his wife, Klaus started psychoanalytic treatment.

During the fifteenth month of his psychoanalysis, Klaus discussed two circumstances reflecting his adolescence passage trauma when his father unexpectedly turned on the light in the family bedroom and the young Klaus caught a glimpse of his mother's vagina. Let us recall that after this bedroom episode he had repeatedly measured the distance between his and his parents' bed, reflecting his desire to be near his mother, but in a concomitant defensive effort, far enough away from her. As an adult, Klaus became an engineer, a surveyor who measured distances. We might say that this aspect of his defensive response to his incestuous desires, contaminated with fear, had become sublimated and adaptive. He grew up to measure distances for a living, so to speak.

The second circumstance stemming from his trauma related to Klaus's conscious fantasy of inventing something that would bring sunlight to the dark side of the Earth during the night hours. His fantasies included thoughts of a spaceship with a vast mirror that would reflect the sun shining on one side of the globe to its dark side. We can see in this a repetition of aspects of the bedroom episode: Klaus would lighten up the darkness and thus see his mother's vagina, but at the same time his defense against incestuous wishes prevailed and kept him from anxiety since it was completely evident that he would never be able to bring light to the darkness.

During the psychoanalytic hours that followed, Klaus was able to express more material regarding his original childhood wishes. He was becoming more and more preoccupied with me and fantasized about triangular situations involving both he and I, along with my secretary, whom he once saw when he came to my office. Klaus's transference neurosis ripened. Soon he began dating a secretary as a displacement for my secretary. It was around this time that he became involved in an unusual activity.

Klaus had found an advertisement in a magazine telling where to find the material for a Viking ship model. He was like a child whose eye had been caught by a toy in a shop window. Should he buy the material for building a Viking ship, or shouldn't he? I did not interfere. After a month or so, Klaus came to a decision and sent for the material. It was an expensive undertaking. When the material arrived, he behaved as if he were a child playing with building blocks. He filled his psychoanalytic hours with accounts of his work with the model. As Klaus planned aloud the next step of his construction, I felt in a pleasant way like a spectator, as if I were watching a son in serious play. Then I observed that Klaus was launching forth into some original creativity beyond what was indicated in the instructions. He wanted to add a lantern that would blink, alternating the light with darkness. Although he was not initially aware of it, his addition would connect him with his trauma at the age of twelve. I wanted to wait and see where Klaus would go with his plan to add a lantern to his Viking ship. He also planned on putting an extra toilet in the model, a toilet suitable for use by a woman.

The ship model had a feminine shape, and through Klaus's measuring and remeasuring its narrow length, it became obvious it represented his mother's vagina. The head of a dragon he used for a figurehead on the prow was the father getting ready to possess the mother and lead her away from the boy. The blinking lantern recalled the bedroom disclosure when Klaus was twelve, as did the toilet designed for a woman. Klaus was concerned over where to put the women's toilet in a ship so narrow. The manufacturer's plans made no allowance for anything but a common toilet. It could be seen that by trying to add a toilet for women only, Klaus was trying to gratify his wish to separate his father's penis from his mother's vagina. He was concerned that it be situated in a place in the ship where no one would see a woman urinating. His desire and dread about seeing his mother's vagina was also repeated here.

Klaus spent nearly $10,000 building his ship. At that time, decades ago, this was a great deal of money. The model was just a showpiece and could not be used on water. Should I have interfered with his therapeutic play from the beginning when he talked about the money needed to build the ship and about his seemingly realistic need to use this amount of money for practical things in his life? Should I have made "interpretations" as he noticed the meanings of various parts of the project such as his adding a blinking lantern? Instead, I waited for Klaus to finish his project. Interestingly, as soon as he finished the Viking ship model with his own modifications, Klaus himself became curious about what he had done. Both Klaus and I verbalized how he had created his mother's vagina, took control as to when a light should shine on it, and how a woman would be separated from a man and have her own privacy.

After his therapeutic play, Klaus reported feeling very different and confident. The Viking ship was no longer important to him. No longer was he interested in my "woman," the secretary. I observed how Klaus began to identify openly with an analytic attitude and became curious about how he had repeated the trauma of age twelve in many, many ways, including his playing a role in pushing his ex-wife to have an affair with his older partner.

CHAPTER 16

Personality organizations

W hen a psychoanalytic clinician meets someone who is seeking treatment, the diagnosis of the person's personality organization is also necessary. Specific types of personality organization play a role in the clinical manifestations of transference, for example, the point at which transference becomes "hot" and the manner in which transference plays its role in the working through of mental conflicts and/or in repairing ego defects. Personality organizations produce some "common" transference as well as countertransference responses. For example, neurotic individuals will primarily focus on issues dealing with the oedipal conflict and defenses and resistances related to such issues. A person with exaggerated narcissism from the beginning of his or her treatment may perceive himself or herself as grandiose while devaluing the therapist. Another individual with exaggerated narcissism may idealize the therapist along with the idealization of himself or herself while constantly devaluing another object.

The diagnosis of personality organization is made by assessing the nature of the patient's self- and object images rather than simply referring to symptoms or character traits and by taking into consideration two ego functions: differentiation and integration. These two ego functions are distinct from encapsulation and externalization, and before focusing on differentiation and integration we will describe and distinguish encapsulation and externalization.

Encapsulation and externalization

The concept of encapsulation describes separating and isolating a traumatized self-image from? its corresponding object images and affects and/or the part of oneself that is a reservoir of tasks given to them by traumatized people from previous generation(s) from the rest of the self-representation (D. Rosenfeld, 1992; H. Rosenfeld, 1965; V. D. Volkan, 1976, 2010). In a sense, encapsulation "splits" the traumatized part of the self-representation and the corresponding object images from the rest of the self-representation and non-conflict-inducing object images. However, such a "splitting" process has not been generalized. Externalizing aspects of oneself to another person or to the external world is similar to Melanie Klein's (1946) concept of "projective identification" (Novick & Kelly, 1970).

Case example of encapsulation and externalization

For instance, Arnold, under the influence of his unconscious fantasy of entering his mother's belly and "killing" his unborn sibling, had become an explorer of caves. Not finding his sibling in the caves, Arnold entered them again and again in various locations. This safeguarded him from the psychic "reality" that he might be a "murderer." After safely exploring a cave, he would function as a "normal" individual, but after some time elapsed, he had to repeat the exploration of the same or another cave so that he could feel "normal" again. In a sense, now and then he visited his "encapsulated" traumatized self, with its own wishes and defenses, as well as the traumatizing object (sibling in the mother's belly). The rest of the time, however, Arnold was "normal" since the traumatizing object did not appear in the caves he explored.

If encapsulation breaks down, the rest of the individual's self-system will be assaulted by the previously encapsulated part and the individual will experience anxiety and confusion. One day, Arnold found an actual dead body while exploring a cave and this broke down his ability to "encapsulate." He became extremely anxious, depressed, and paranoid. He had to be hospitalized.

Differentiation, integration, developmental splitting, defensive splitting

Above we have described the levels of separation–individuation. A person who cannot go through the separation–individuation phases in a normal fashion will have difficulties as an adult in testing reality and knowing and sensing how different objects have their own boundaries. Also, until a child can tolerate ambivalence, there is a "normal" developmental splitting of opposing self- and object images. Later, a child begins to bring opposing images together. Those who cannot achieve such a melding of opposite images to one degree or other turn their previous developmental splitting into a *defensive splitting*.

Four personality organizations

Here we will list four personality organizations according to their ability to perform differentiation and integration.

They are:

1. *Neurotic* personality organization
2. *Narcissistic* personality organization
3. *Borderline* personality organization
4. *Psychotic* personality organization.

In fact, the list of personality organizations is longer if we consider the fact that the organizations listed above can be divided into subgroups when we observe the nature of unconscious fantasies attached to them and/or the nature of symptom manifestations reflecting the dominance of a part of the internal structure expressing itself outwardly. For example, we consider the personality organization of a neurotic patient with a typical unconscious fantasy that stays within the psychological realm to be different from the personality organization of another neurotic individual with an "actualized" or "concretized" unconscious fantasy that, when it is activated, causes serious difficulty in the individual's ability to separate where the fantasy starts and where the reality begins.

There are also different types of narcissistic personality organizations. Arnold Cooper (1989) described a type of narcissistic personality organization that urges the individual toward repeating masochistic behavior in order to feel special and secretly grandiose. Patients with this type of narcissistic personality organization make their suffering "ego-syntonic": "I am the one who forced my mother to be cruel. I like to be frustrated" (p. 549). Cooper added that such persons "are masochistically unwilling to end their feelings of deprivation, and their narcissism required that they not relinquish the sense that they have suffered specially, and that special reparations are due to them" (p. 550).

Also, we can consider a *multiple personality organization* (I. Brenner, 2001, 2004) that refers to various and rather formed but unintegrated internal structures (self-images or a combination of self- and object images) expressing themselves outwardly, each at different times and each with its own "identity," as a subgroup either of a borderline or of a psychotic personality organization. In fact, we may consider dissociative personality organization as a separate internal structure.

Case example of neurotic transference and transference neurosis

George, a physician in his mid-thirties with an obsessional character, went into treatment because of his puzzlement and distress over his wife's leaving him. It became clear during the therapeutic process that he had been a virtual slave to his wife during their seven years of marriage. He had gone out of his way to please her, giving her gifts he could ill afford; doing the dishes and emptying the garbage when he had no time for such chores; rubbing her back to help her sleep when his hands were tired, and so on. Underneath all this compliant behavior smoldered silent hostility and denial of his dependence on a woman.

George's mother, an adopted child, had clung to a fantasy that she had originally been born into a noble family. When George was born to her, she conveyed to him her passion to be recognized as glorious and expected him to realize her fantasy by attaining great fame. Her attitude accounted in some measure for her son's behaving as a slave to please women, including his ex-wife, and his continued resentment of them.

George's already stressed relationship with his mother had an added complication when he reached the oedipal age. His mother was in the habit of leaving her husband's bed during the night and wandering from room to room of the house, going bed to bed. This awakened in the oedipal boy fantasies about claiming her from his father, whom his mother often disparaged in his presence. The growing boy took secret pride in his belief that he would surpass his father and become not only a better man than he but one more greatly loved by his mother. He could not escape the idea, however, that his father would punish him for having such oedipal-incestuous wishes. His father often beat little George for behavior that offended his mother since this behavior expressed the child's wish to be free of her. On these occasions, George had to bend over before his father and allow himself to be struck.

A year after George began his psychoanalytic treatment, it seemed that his incestuous wishes in boyhood had barely been repressed; since childhood, whenever he had masturbated, he had often fantasized about a sexual encounter with his mother. Soon after entering puberty, George amputated his toe "accidentally," and his dreams showed that this was an act of self-castration to foil any castration his father might attempt. His self-castration helped him to repress his fear of his father. However, this fear was betrayed in certain fantasies. For example, as an adult, he would fantasize that the husband or lover of any woman in whom he felt an interest would meet with an automobile accident and die. Then on many occasions he himself would have an accident in his car.

George's father died of cancer soon after his son's marriage, and at the moment of his death, the younger couple were having intercourse in the room just below the death chamber. George's association to this led him to understand that he wanted to have sex with his wife while his father was dying and that this act primarily was designed to show the dying man that his son now had his own woman and had no interest in his father's wife (George's own mother). At one level, it was his wish to resolve his Oedipus complex magically just before his father died by, in a sense, saying to the old man, "See, I have my woman and you have your woman, my mother. Both of us are men with their own women. There is no need for a competition and there is no need for a murder or castration."

At the beginning of the third year of his psychoanalysis, George's realization of his magical wish to resolve his oedipal conflict quickly, and his deeper and emotional understanding of his unresolved oedipal conflict allowed him to feel closer to the image of his father. In turn, he could now mourn over losing him. I was moved to see this obsessional individual weep very genuinely for his father's death on the couch after two years of treatment.

After his mourning over his father, in the third year of his analysis, George could bring his oedipal struggle in full force to his psychoanalysis and develop a full-blown transference neurosis. In the transference, I became the oedipal father. George became involved with the secretary of another psychiatrist, who appeared in his dreams wearing a moustache. I had a moustache at that time, but my colleague did not: George was fusing the other psychiatrist with me into one image. When I did not say anything and waited for the transference to become a workable transference neurosis, George gave up the affair and began clearly disparaging me during his sessions. At the same time, he also feared me. Again, I did not interfere.

Then George began to have a ritual during his sessions: before lying down, he would sit on the couch and remove his contact lenses. After the session was over once more, he would sit on the couch and replace the lenses before leaving. In a sense he was symbolically plucking out his eyes (self-castration, not unlike his having an accident and losing his toe) so he would not be castrated—because he was already castrated. I did nothing about this ritual until George had a dream in which he attacked a representation of me, which was still another psychiatrist, while forgetting to remove his contact lenses before the fight and injuring his cornea. George felt anxiety on my couch and then I told him what I understood about his ritual. After this, George stopped his ritual but had fantasies of a miracle cure that would restore his eyes to 20/20 vision. Again, he would magically undo his castration. When this was interpreted, he began experiencing more "naked" oedipal struggles.

George wanted to be hypnotized so he could open his "memory box," and when I interpreted that he wanted me to "move into him" by means of hypnosis, he came up with the idea that I had a curved penis; I was a terrible Turk with a scimitar (curved penis) with which to decapitate people. George blanched and shook with anxiety on my couch. Then recalling that he himself had a curved penis, he thought I must have a double curve, and finally, after some weeks, he decided that mine had the shape of the letter S. For him, S stood not only for "snake," but also for "shit," an anal phase symbol.

George recalled defecating on the living room floor at the age of four and seeing the family dog eat his excrement. He recalled his amazement, delight, and fear over this episode with affect. "Shit is powerful," he remarked. I told him to consider the idea that if one eats the bodily material or body part of another, one can steal the other's characteristics, such as power. This led to George's fellatio fantasies, and he talked about his realization that he wanted to eat my penis. He talked about such fantasies for days and shook with anxiety while I stayed silent most of the time, allowing him to experience and own his castration anxiety. Soon George was able to report "good" things about his father, and to realize his anger toward his mother for keeping him, as he felt, from being friendly with his father. Then, slowly he began to feel friendly toward me. He was on his way to working through his Oedipus complex.

What George had done can easily be explained by the classical descriptions of transference and transference neurosis. George owned the opposing aspects of his conflicts within himself, especially after some previously unconscious aspects of his conflicts were brought to his attention. This vignette shows that the transference neurosis is a new "version" of a patient's neurosis; in it, the analyst becomes the focal figure upon whom conflicts between instinctual drives and defenses against them, originally a part of childhood experience, are displaced. The feelings a patient experiences during transference neurosis are uniquely vivid in the present, so upon being interpreted they become authentic for him or her. The patient feels convinced of the relevance of interpretations and his understanding of what he has been repeating in the analyst's office.

Here we present another of Vamık Volkan's cases to illustrate a narcissistic transference turning into a neurotic transference.

Case example of a narcissistic transference

Brown was thirty years old when his psychoanalysis started. He was a man who viewed himself as the center of the world and believed that he was superior to others. For example, during summers, he would go to a swimming pool at a country club and sit by the pool in his swimming suit and imagine that everybody was looking at him and admiring him.

He and his wife had two daughters. When his wife gave birth to their third child, a boy, there was some question at birth about the baby's health. He might not grow up to be physically "perfect." One of Brown's maternal ancestors had been a colonial leader, playing an important role in the birth of the United States. Brown felt that his frail son damaged the "specialness" of the family name. Brown's self-esteem was threatened. Accordingly, soon after his son's birth, he seduced a judge's daughter. This woman worked as a secretary at a prestigious law firm. Brown's father was the head of the law firm, and had employed Brown to work there. According to Brown, his affair with the judge's daughter was a "wonderful" love affair. However, she became pregnant, had an abortion, and the affair ended. It was at this point that Brown became very anxious and sought treatment.

On the surface, Brown's affair with a judge's daughter who was a secretary at Brown's father's firm appeared to be related to oedipal concerns. What comes to mind is this: having an "imperfect" child (representing his penis) reactivated Brown's castration anxiety and in turn, he seduced a woman who "belonged" to his father or a judge in order to have an oedipal triumph. The woman represented a mother figure. Paradoxically, his attempt to have an oedipal triumph and this woman's aborting a fetus increased Brown's castration anxiety. After Brown's analysis started, I learned that oedipal issues were *not* "hot" in Brown's mind.

Brown's main concern was to protect an internal aspect of himself that is known in the psychoanalytic literature as a "grandiose self." This term was first used by Heinz Kohut (1971). He referred to children's searching for perfection and its fixation in some adults. Later, Otto Kernberg (1975) also used the same term to describe the pathological internal structure in some adults that was formed to maintain good aspects of childhood, an idealized self-image that protects the person from feeling upset and angry, and a fantasized ever-loving parent.

Having an "imperfect" child was a blow to Brown's grandiose self, and to reestablish this self he had chosen a special lover. The judge's daughter, as was learned by him *only* during the second year of his analysis, was "a mess." She was not pretty, and she had an abdominal tumor that once removed left ugly scars on her body. She was a kleptomaniac. She had had problems with her teeth, which were removed and replaced with false teeth.

I imagined that this woman removed her false teeth while performing fellatio on Brown and that this helped to ease Brown's fear of a *vagina dentata*. However, during the initial years of his psychoanalysis, his primary focus was not on psychosexual issues. Instead, Brown had used this woman to feed his grandiose self. Throughout the affair, in his mind, he constantly compared himself physically and mentally with his lover so he could easily feel that he was the superior one. His lover helped him to maintain his grandiose self.

Now I will tell the story of some aspects of Brown's "narcissistic transference." Brown started his analysis with a monotonous voice, giving forth endless accounts that seemed designed less as communication to the analyst than as productions to elicit wonder. The first obvious transference manifestation occurred a few weeks after his analysis started. He flew to a resort where he seduced a "foreign woman" who spoke English with an accent (I am Turkish. I migrated to the United States, thus I was a "foreigner" and like this woman, spoke English with an accent). Brown had no warmth toward this woman. He "screwed" and devalued her. In this transference-related act, Brown repeated finding a "lower" status person, comparing himself with the devalued one, coming out on top, and feeding his grandiose self.

During the initial years of Brown's psychoanalysis, I learned the reasons why Brown had developed a narcissistic personality organization. He had a rather typical childhood history that supports the development of such an organization (Kernberg, 1975; V. D. Volkan, 2010; V. D. Volkan & Ast, 1994). There was a cold mother who failed to give him adequate love, while passing him a sense that he was born to be "special," which was an extension of her famous colonial leader ancestor. The father was aloof. As a child, Brown was left alone to constantly daydream. (Here I will refrain from giving the specifics of his traumatic childhood story or any details of the technique of treating such an individual, for example, allowing the narcissistic transference time to fully develop. I will simply focus on a description of the nature of his transference and its developing story.)

During the initial years on the couch, Brown did not experience anxiety or frustration for long; he became a push-button man, handling his anxiety and frustration by summoning up a daydream or fantasy that would support his grandiosity as though pushing a television control, while believing that his analysis would be a "smashing success."

As time passed, Brown gave names to his fantasies on the couch such as "iron ball," "bountiful woman," and "raped girl." Lying on the couch, he would simply say he had had—or, he was having—another of his so-and-so fantasies. The "iron ball" was a rather typical "glass bubble fantasy" (K. Volkan, 2021a; V. D. Volkan, 1979, 2010) in that a patient with a narcissistic personality organization lives alone in a fantastic kingdom while keeping others away. The "bountiful woman" fantasy described his finding an idealized woman who unconditionally loved and fed him. The "raped girl" fantasy reflected variations of his actual relationship with the judge's daughter.

Case example of developing a neurotic transference

Brown brought in a brand new daydream and called it a "Henry VIII" fantasy. At this time, he was reading a book on Henry VIII. The English king represented Brown's symbol of his own grandiosity since Brown's colonial ancestor is of British origin. Henry VIII was a fat person and thus he also represented Brown's babyhood "bad" mother, who had become obese when Brown was a baby. In his daydream, Brown was in England as a leader of a democratic colony newly formed under the aegis of a "foreign power" (the analyst as a "new object") that was designed to bring an easygoing democratic lifestyle to England. The term "new object" sometimes is called "developmental object" or "analytic object" (Cameron, 1961; Giovacchini, 1972; Kernberg, 1975; Loewald, 1960; Tähkä, 1993; V. D. Volkan, 1976; V. D. Volkan & Ast, 1992, 1994). This new image is differentiated from the patient's archaic images that are displaced onto the analyst as part of transference manifestations. The patient's experiences with such an object and identifications with its function would allow him or her to begin to integrate images in his or her internal world.

In the book Brown was reading, he had noted a footnote about the Turks (me) that indicated their power at the time and described their onslaught at the gates of Vienna. Brown acknowledged my "power," rendered it a "benign power," and used this success to tame his grandiose self and the image of his "fat mother." In his daydream, he captured Henry VIII and imprisoned him and felt that the tyrannical king was safely away.

The next day, Brown continued to understand other meanings of his dream. He thought that Henry VIII, ever overeating and thus obese, not only represented his grandiose self but his devalued (hungry for love) aspects that he had put on people like the judge's daughter or in the transference, on me, and that he had kept split-off from his grandiose self. His Henry VIII daydream thus represented a "crucial juncture" in that he brought together his grandiose and hungry self-images. Thus, he began to have a cohesive self-representation and moved up to a neurotic personality organization.

Only after evolving a neurotic personality organization was Brown able to experience the oedipal and other psychosexual aspects of his affair with the judge's daughter. The "iron ball" no longer referred to his grandiose kingdom but to his testicles. When he had a narcissistic personality organization, he believed that he had the best sexual organs. Now, he noticed that one scrotal sac was smaller than the other. He actually went to see a physician (again representing me), who examined his "balls," told him that testes were normally unequal in size, and reassured him that he was a normal and "average" man.

In Brown's case, the transference he exhibited during the initial years forces us to expand the classical description of this concept. Brown did not experience his hungry and devalued part as belonging to himself; often he behaved as if his analyst were a "nothing," without being aware that the analyst represented his devalued images. Only in the fourth year of his analysis was Brown able to let me into his previously lonely but glorious kingdom. He then owned his opposing images, integrated my representation, and in turn became a normal "average" individual.

Case example of a borderline transference

Saul was not a typical person with a borderline personality organization who comes to analysis or whom psychoanalysts easily accept to analyze.

Here we recount the story of his "split transference" because no other patient in our experience ever exhibited this type of transference and its hierarchical evolution as concretely as Saul (V. D. Volkan, 1976).

When Saul was a child, he sat at a corner and rocked himself and appeared in a dream state. He would not answer when he was spoken to. His entire vocabulary at age four consisted of six words: "hi," "mama," "dada," "candy," "bacon," and "bye-bye." He did not start talking until he was six years old. When he was a child, his parents took him to see Leo Kanner. Saul was one of the kids Leo Kanner (1894–1981) studied. These studies, along with Hans Asperger's work, represent the modern studies on what is generally known as "autism," or as it was sometimes called, the "Kanner syndrome" (Kanner, 1942).

Saul's parents were rich and were determined that their son would get any treatment that might help him. So, Saul was sent to special schools and was subjected to various behavior modification techniques. At the end, in his late teens, he was sent to the then well-known Chestnut Lodge Hospital. He spent some years there both as an inpatient and an outpatient and received individual psychoanalytically oriented therapy. Through this, it was possible that he was able to consolidate his inner world at a borderline personality organization level. Later, he was sent for psychoanalysis to help him to move up on the developmental ladder. He was seen on the couch four times a week for more than five years.

When Saul started psychoanalysis, he had just become a student at the University of Virginia. During puberty, and thereafter, Saul had studied mathematics, physics, astronomy, and other fields of learning that required no social interaction and lacked emotional content. He had begun thinking of himself as a "genius," and was encouraged to do so by his mother. Nevertheless, his self-representation as an idiot persisted.

He also divided his object images as genius or idiot. When he came to the University of Virginia, other than routine daily interactions that involved making purchases and providing for himself, he lived for all intents and purposes a solitary life. He had a naive regard for his few "friends," who, in his view, could suddenly change into "all bad" people. He judged others according to his estimate of their IQ. This was the only dimension of others that was meaningful to Saul. He was overweight and walked like a penguin. He came to his sessions with greasy pants and often he stuffed toilet tissue in his shirt pockets and under his shirt. Sometimes toilet paper hung out from his sleeves.

Saul was able to express that his mother was intrusive in promoting his bowel training. When he was a child, she gave him an enema at any sign of constipation from the time he was a year and a half old. Soon it was possible to make a formulation as Saul's early life became apparent. His Jewish father had fled Europe as a boy and made a fortune collecting and selling scrap metal. The father was not an educated person. When he was forty years old, the father married a musically talented woman from a very small town. She was a college graduate, a Christian, and about twenty years younger than Saul's father. This woman was frustrated and remorseful because she believed that she could have been a great pianist if she had not married an older man from a different culture and religion. She secretly felt superior in culture and education to her husband. In her mind, he was just an ignorant man who had made a fortune by collecting and selling others' garbage. This was a secret "split" in the family. Her first son belonged to her husband. She wanted Saul, her second son, to be hers and to be her extension. By giving the boy frequent enemas, she wanted him to be clean and superior, not contaminated with "garbage."

The first visible transference manifestation of Saul was his perceiving me to be like his mother. The toilet tissues suggested that he was ready to be cleaned and thus to please his analyst/mother who was "all good" and a genius. But during the first year of his treatment, Saul could not pronounce the word "enema." Instead of "enema" he would say something like "anemia." This gave the sense that the intrusion of the mother also made her image one of a blood-sucking caretaker. The "all good" image of the mother was split off from the "all bad" image of the mother. Saul, in his sessions, was either a "genius" or an "idiot." For him, there was no concept of being average.

Before reporting a story of Saul's attempt to mend his and others' split images in the transference, we have some general comments about the treatment of such an individual. If we read the psychoanalytic literature on the treatment of people suffering from borderline personality disorder, we notice that there are two methods of approach.

The first technique aims to keep the patient at the level at which he or she is already functioning but strives to circumvent further regression by providing new "ego experiences" through clarifications, suggestions, confrontations, and interpretations. These can help the patient integrate opposing self- as well as object representations. Psychoanalysts who endorse this style of treatment for borderline personality disorder maintain that if their already undeveloped and regressed patients regress further, they will become psychotic and lose the ability to differentiate self- and object images and thus be unable to test reality.

Proponents of the second and perhaps more difficult approach, elaborated by Vamık Volkan (1987, 2010), maintain that patients with borderline personality organization must experience further regression to truly modify their inner structure. This regression is therapeutically controlled. The idea of regression giving way to a new psychic organization has been demonstrated in the developmental process and under certain clinical conditions. For example, in normal development, a new psychic organization is ushered in by the natural regression that takes place during adolescence (Blos, 1966, 1979); in uncomplicated mourning, after the loss of a love object, the mourner experiences regression before being able to reestablish an adaptation to his or her external reality and his or her inner world.

In controlled therapeutic regression, an individual with a borderline personality organization can abandon the *defensive* use of splitting and reactivate "normal" *developmental* splitting. Once the patient is back on his or her developmental course, the patient can follow the path of psychic growth and gain integrative ego ability, just as a child would. Psychoanalysts who advocate this approach know that transference psychosis may accompany the therapeutic regression, and they are willing to continue analytic work if it does.

In Saul's case, he would speak as if he was a superman when he was on the couch. He spoke like a genius about galaxies while he mocked others. During other sessions, he was an "idiot." Sometimes he made me an extension of his genius image, and other times I joined his idiot image. At times, he simply rocked on the couch. Developing various and bizarre cannibalistic fantasies, Saul was able to regress therapeutically, especially during the second year of his psychoanalytic work. Saul had masturbation fantasies of sucking up his mother's image into his chest and hearing his mother's orders as inner hallucinations. Later in his "transference psychosis", he sucked me up through his penis. Saul's image fused with the image of me. Saul slowly began to differentiate his self-image from his mother's and my images.

Case example of a "crucial juncture" experience

Soon Saul began coming to his appointments twenty-five minutes late. At the time, my analytic office was at the University of Virginia Hospital. The door of my office opened to a hallway. Typically, the office door would be left open for patients to walk in. Upon entering my room, patients would close the door behind them and take their place on the couch. After coming in twenty-five minutes late, Saul would have a big smile on his face and with enthusiasm would quickly lie on my couch and say: "And, another thing, doctor," and give a report on some event. I would feel elated about Saul's enthusiasm and experience pleasure of his being on the couch. In other words, Saul was "good," and the analyst was also "good." By saying, "And, another thing, doctor," Saul was creating a continuity between his last session, where Saul and I were both "good", and the current session.

I became curious about why Saul had begun coming to each session twenty-five minutes late. It seemed intellectually that Saul was splitting the sessions between myself and himself by being absent during the first half of his hour and present in the second. I did not try to interfere and waited to see what would develop while this went on for about a month. When asked if he was aware of coming to his sessions in the middle of his hours, Saul responded with a big grin and said: "You are all wrong, doctor." He was in such a good mood that I also had a grin on my face sitting behind him.

I eventually learned that Saul indeed came on time but spent the first twenty-five minutes of his assigned hour on the toilet in a bathroom next door. While there, he imagined me to be a monster, an enema-giving and blood-sucking intrusive mother. My "all bad" image was in the bathroom separated (split) from my office by a wall. While in the office, Saul deposited an "all good" parent image into me and made me feel "elated." Saul, in a concrete way, was experiencing a splitting of his and my self-representations. In the transference, Saul made me a partner in his activities and feelings. I hoped that this was to be a clear indication of his starting "developmental splitting." I also hoped that in the future, Saul would bring his opposing aspects together, initially in a "crucial juncture" experience. After this session, Saul resumed coming on time to his sessions. The term "crucial juncture" was first used by Melanie Klein (1946). It refers to a patient's experiences in the service of bringing together his or her opposite self- and object images so that he or she could begin to mend his or her internal world.

Saul's "crucial juncture" experience was concrete and dramatic. One day, during a routine and comfortable analytic session, Saul suddenly got up from the couch and physically attacked me. The attack was surprising. I defended myself and no one was hurt. Saul seemed to be flooded with emotions for several minutes when he had "contact" with me. He also seemed surprised. Saul left the room—perhaps to retreat to the bathroom. However, he soon returned, apologized like a grown-up person with a clear voice, and took his place on the couch. The rest of this session and some of his future sessions were spent analyzing his surprise attack and his having physical contact with me.

Some technical mistake or unconscious action of mine may have provoked this incident. However, on reflection, this was not apparent. Trying to collect Saul's associations of his physical contact with me, I realized that the incident represented a "crucial juncture" experience. Saul, as an "old bad" image, was making a contact with me as an "all good" image. This, as he sensed, was the first experience for him of this kind. Saul's experience of being flooded with emotions during this incident represented a primitive anxiety about mending opposing images. We can put ourselves in a child's place and imagine experiencing panic about "losing" our "all good" aspect when a mending of opposites begins to take place.

Soon after this incident, Saul began attending meetings at a Christian resort, "The Bridge," a meeting place for people to find salvation through religion. It seemed that the name of this organization attracted him to this place. The name, The Bridge, reflected his continuing attempt to create a link between his opposing self- and object images. Since Saul was like a developing child, and moving from developmental splitting to a cohesive self-representation as well as cohesive representations of others, there was no reason to "interpret" the meaning of his activity.

I was like a child analyst watching and guiding a young person in going through normal developmental stages.

Saul learned how to meet and to know other persons by going to The Bridge. Soon he began going into a courthouse a few times a week, where he sat through trials in order, as he reported, "to learn about human beings." He was also prompted to sit closer to his classmates without stuffing his shirt pocket and under his shirt with toilet tissues, and began losing his obesity.

He had a dream of being in a hallway leading to four locations: a cafeteria, a barbershop, a bookstore, and a post office. Saul said that the cafeteria was his mother, the barbershop was his father, and the bookstore was himself. He thought that I was the post office since I was making him a male (mail) and sending him, like an envelope to new (psychic) locations. The interesting thing in the dream was that Saul saw himself moving his bowels without embarrassment in the hallway. In the dream, Saul felt that he demonstrated autonomy in moving his bowels without a need for an enema. Next, he began to show interest in me as a father figure. He stopped going to the Christian place, The Bridge, and began visiting the campus organization, Hillel. It should be recalled that Saul's father was Jewish.

Much, much later, many years after his analysis was finished, at an airport, running from one gate to another, I bumped into Saul. We were surprised at meeting each other this way. Saul said that he had become a psychologist and that he was teaching at a university.

Saul's case illustrates defensive splitting turning into developmental splitting. Here, the transference story reflects self-disturbance and the need to develop new ego functions to repair this disturbance and develop an ability to have cohesive self- and object images and representations. To develop new ego functions, Saul took his analyst in through his penis during his therapeutic regression, slowly changed what he had taken into a "new object" (Loewald, 1960), and identified with it and its ego functions for mental growth.

CHAPTER 17

A story of a psychoanalysis illustrating psychoanalytic terms and concepts

In this chapter, we recount the first fourteen months of treatment of Vamık Volkan's analysand, who was exiled as a child and who fought in Vietnam as an adult. The aim here is to illustrate some psychoanalytic concepts mentioned above, such as not having a good enough mother, separation–individuation problems, activities reflecting oedipal fantasies, traumas in childhood, and traumas in adulthood. We will also describe the analysand's defense mechanisms, including encapsulations, and linking childhood traumas and fantasies to actions in a war zone in adulthood, and the psychoanalytic clinician's experience holding on to his or her therapeutic identity while listening to horrible stories. This psychoanalytic story starts with the observation of a built-in transference and ends with a dream that shows how the patient gained a major insight about his internal world.

Case example of Alfonso

Alfonso, a handsome man, was thirty-nine years old when he began working with me in the late 1990s. He is the firstborn child of Catholic Portuguese immigrants to the United States, who lived in a community of people of Portuguese descent in New York City. When Alfonso's parents married, his mother was thirty years old and his father was thirty-seven years old. Alfonso's father had arrived in the United States from Portugal as a young man and therefore spoke English with a heavy accent. One year after their marriage, Alfonso was born.

Before Alfonso's birth, his father was gone overseas, serving as a United States World War II soldier although never seeing any combat. During that time, the child was cared for by his mother and maternal grandmother, the latter dying when Alfonso was three years old. Alfonso does not have memories of his grandmother. He was told however that his grandmother, like his father, was an immigrant from Portugal who spoke English with a heavy accent, and that she was a strict person who slapped Alfonso's mother even after she was mature and demanded obedience.

While pregnant with Alfonso, his mother fell and was bedridden for some months. She was cared for by her mother and other female relatives in the Portuguese immigrant community where they lived. A difficult delivery with forceps caused her a painful urinary infection and Alfonso's mother would repeat the story of her travail repeatedly, telling her son, "You are alive because of me." Alfonso's mother overfed her infant son. As the boy grew, she was also seductive and interested in her son's bodily functions, especially his toilet training.

Later in Alfonso's psychoanalysis, I would learn more about Alfonso's mother's reaction formation, changing unacceptable to acceptable. Instead of holding on to her frustration for not having her husband around during her pregnancy and responding to her physical difficulties while pregnant and while delivering Alfonso, she "loved" her son by becoming an intrusive mother.

When Alfonso's father returned from World War II, the boy was almost four years old. He felt anxious being in the same room alone with his father, who, as I learned later, was not punitive. But Alfonso sensed that his father was trying to break up the "intimacy" between mother and son by encouraging him to go out into the streets to play with other boys, although the neighborhood was a rough one. Alfonso's father did not wish to have a "sissy child" who clung to his mother.

When Alfonso was six years old, his sister was born. Alfonso was then sent in a propeller-driven airplane with a female, teenage chaperone to Portugal to live with his paternal grandmother and other relatives. The airplane ride took many hours and as the plane shook in the air, he felt that he might die. The boy was not prepared for this separation and felt very confused, rejected, and helpless. After his arrival in rural Portugal, he packed his suitcase every day with the idea that he would be taken back to his mother. But six months passed before he was allowed to return to his paternal home. While in Portugal, he felt as if he were "exiled" without even knowing intellectually what this word means. His pre-oedipal separation–individuation problems related to his mother and his oedipal expectation of punishment by his father were actualized in his mind.

When he returned to the United States, he found his mother busy with his sister, whom he hated and continued to hate. He was also angry at his mother, who first intensely "loved" him and then sent him away and abandoned him. Now, Alfonso wanted very badly to reestablish his special relationship with his mother. The more he wanted his mother, the more he became afraid of his father. He also felt embarrassed by his father because of the older man's emotionalism and heavy accent. However, in his daily life he smiled at his parents and appeared to be a good boy; meanwhile, he was fascinated with movies about the Wild West, shooting Indians, and dueling between "good" and "evil" cowboys.

When he became an adolescent, at the age of twelve, his father gave Alfonso a gift of a rifle, and demanded that the boy study rules for gun safety. Soon after this, Alfonso took the rifle into the family room to show it to friends. Resenting his mother's reference to this as dangerous, he said: "I know what I am doing." Then he pointed his gun at her and pulled the trigger, sending a bullet into the wall behind her; it seemed a miracle that she had not been killed. He reported having sunk to the floor afterwards. Then, with the help of his mother, he patched the hole in the wall; neither ever spoke of this event to Alfonso's father.

As a teenager, Alfonso masturbated daily. He knew that his mother at times watched him through the keyhole of his bedroom, as she had also done when he was a small boy. His mother would examine his bed sheets to see if he had soiled the linen through masturbation. But she would never tell him, "Stop masturbating," and they would never talk about his masturbation out in the open.

Between the ages of twelve and fourteen, he stole condoms that belonged to his father from a drawer in the parental bedroom. Alfonso put them on his penis and masturbated while thinking of making love to his mother. At the same time, he would be petrified when his father returned home from work. He thought that his father would count his condoms, find out that some were missing, and become angry and punish him. In a sense, he brought his oedipal wishes and fears to life during his adolescence passage.

Alfonso became preoccupied with imaginary "intruders" as a teenager. He felt that some persons would forcibly enter their house and punish or kill him. At the same time, he was conscious of his wish that his father be dead. On the surface, he continued to idealize his mother and behave like an obedient young man. Internally, however, things were becoming unbearable. So, in his late teens he found an older married woman (an obvious mother substitute) and became her lover, eventually moving in with her. This woman's husband was a criminal but locked up in a prison, so Alfonso knew that he was dangerous.

Alfonso's mother disapproved of him moving in with his older, married lover. But Alfonso continued to live with this woman for about two years. This arrangement at first appeared to be workable. But one day, his lover's little boy began calling Alfonso "Daddy." Alfonso became very anxious, left this woman, and enrolled in the police academy. As a police cadet, Alfonso carried a gun on a belt around his waist and went around with an older policeman catching criminals. But this new "adjustment" was not enough, so Alfonso decided to enlist in the armed forces, and went to Vietnam, where a hellish war was being fought.

In Vietnam, Alfonso eventually became a platoon leader. His platoon's main job was to search for and kill the enemy in the bush or jungle. One day, Alfonso stayed behind while his men went into the bush under the leadership of another platoon leader. That day, his men and their temporary platoon leader were ambushed, and all of them were killed. The corpses were brought to the main camp, and Alfonso went to see their mutilated bodies and experienced extreme survival guilt. His term of service in Vietnam was coming to an end, yet despite this horrific event, he volunteered to serve a second year-long tour of duty in the war zone.

After his two voluntary tours in Vietnam, Alfonso returned to his parents' house. He was still in his twenties, and he lived with his parents for more than a year before getting employment at a big grocery store and moving into his own place. During this time, he developed a new masturbation ritual he nicknamed "risky business." This ritual was as follows: In his parents' absence, he would mount their bed as though he were atop his mother and masturbate while gazing at a picture of her on the bedside table. He then had conscious wishes for his father's death. Once, thinking that thieves had entered the building in which his parents' apartment was located, he went to the window and fired at the people he thought were the fleeing burglars using the same gun given to him by his father when he was twelve years old.

After moving out of his parents' home, Alfonso became a vegetarian, turned to Buddhism and meditation, and embraced celibacy. Some years later he gave up celibacy. The day he did this, Alfonso almost killed himself in a swimming accident, diving into shallow waters and injuring his head and shoulder. Eventually, he went on to study and become a teacher of sociology. He also married a woman who had come to the United States from Sweden and who had become a social worker. Alfonso wanted me to hear that his wife's striking blonde hair contrasted sharply with his mother's darker hair. Alfonso and his family eventually moved away from the area where his parents lived to a location near to the city, where I lived and practiced my profession. Alfonso continued to teach sociology at his new location.

Alfonso maintained ritualistic telephone calls to his mother and told everyone what a great woman he thought she was. He did not communicate directly with his father and very seldom got in touch with his sister, who lived away from the parental home, but within driving distance. Alfonso and his wife had their first child, a boy, and Alfonso developed a good reputation as a sociologist by encapsulating the troubled aspects of his internal world. While he was teaching, he could remain an intellectual person and teacher whose psychological issues were hidden away. When I first saw him, he had been married for nine years, and their son was two years old.

Obviously, I knew nothing about Alfonso's history when I first saw him. His story that I reported above came to my attention slowly. Now, starting with my diagnostic interview, I will repeat what I heard from him as time went on; thus, there will be some repetition of his history. Furthermore, I will report what I thought and what I felt about his remarks and actions. I will also tell you how I responded to him. Alfonso's case brings some very challenging issues to a psychoanalyst's attention.

The diagnostic interview

During our initial interview, Alfonso stated that he was seeking psychoanalysis to understand himself better, and he described his background to me without much detail. He knew that he had chosen to become a sociologist in order to understand his position in society and to know more about himself. He said that his marriage was a good one and that he loved his son. I learned that Alfonso maintained a ritualistic yet distant relationship with his parents and sister. Mother and son would reassure each other of their special, mutual "love" in telephone conversations that Alfonso would cut short whenever his father came to the telephone.

I concluded that despite the stress he placed on his macho image, Alfonso had unresolved oedipal conflicts and sibling rivalry issues. He seemed to use a great deal of intellectualization and other obsessional defenses. I thought that we would be able to work together well. I also thought that his psychoanalysis would be rather routine. Unfortunately, I was unable to fit a new analysand into my schedule at the time. I told Alfonso it would be at least a year before I could do so and suggested that he might want to seek another psychoanalyst. He replied that it would serve him to wait a year and that another year would find him in a better position to financially afford treatment.

A year passed before Alfonso came to start our work together. I remember thinking that one of the reasons he wanted to wait to work with me was the fact that I have an accent when speaking in English. Since I thought that he had unresolved oedipal issues, symbolically I would fit well with the image of his oedipal father, who also spoke English with an accent. In retrospect, I did not conduct a very thorough diagnostic interview. Once his psychoanalysis started, I saw that I had missed some significant factors at our first encounter.

Alfonso's built-in transference

One year after our initial encounter, Alfonso started his psychoanalysis four times a week lying on my couch. He seemed like a different person.

He did not appear to be the polite and intellectual sociologist. At the outset, his dress—khaki trousers, brown shirt, and leather vest—gave the impression of a military uniform. I was puzzled by the intensity of his feelings toward me, his conviction that I was harsh, unempathic, and selfish. He seemed to believe that I would reject him from psychoanalysis no matter what he did.

Although he was preoccupied with his parents, he had not seen them in four years. He applied to his father the same harsh terms he used to describe me, adding that as a youth he could not enter the room in which his father stored the various tools that the old man used, the names of which Alfonso could not remember. He had anxiety about coming to my office. He recalled that as a child, after a day of being his mother's darling, he would flee to his own room upon hearing a rattling keychain announcing his father's arrival home from work. Now, he was afraid that if he made a sound coming into my office I would be disturbed and reject him from psychoanalysis.

Alfonso reported that during the year he awaited psychoanalysis, he had kept a picture of me from one of my books by his bedside and had conversations with it each night. I realized that in my physical absence, he had started his psychoanalysis by himself. During the year before Alfonso started psychoanalytic treatment, there was little influence from reality toward taming his developing transference stories. As such, we had started out with a "built-in transference."

Alfonso felt threatened by my every sound, every utterance, and he responded dramatically like an actor on stage, displaying his muscles and saying, "I'll take whatever you give me," or alternatively bursting into sobs and abruptly suppressing them. I learned to my amazement that during the year he awaited treatment, his wife had attended some of my seminars using her maiden name. Obviously, I did not know that Alfonso's wife was a participant in my seminars. When Alfonso asked about me, she reported to him that I was tough and that I would "tame" him.

I learned that during the year while he had my picture by his bedside, he was celibate, only having some sexual activities while taking showers with his wife. He would reach orgasm when she rubbed his penis. I felt that given the year of his conversations with my picture, contamination of his psychoanalysis by his wife's attendance at my seminars, and his collection of information about me, it might be better that he see another psychoanalyst. Without sharing my thinking with him, I vacillated in my mind as to whether we should continue or not but, in the end, I decided to keep him as an analysand.

I commented on Alfonso's apparent wish to protect himself from me and spoke of his having a "psychoanalysis" with me (with my picture) during the year before he came into actual treatment, suggesting that fantasies about me developed during that period were interfering with our work, since he was only conversing with my picture and I did not know of these fantasies. I then asked to him to consider a fresh start on the real psychoanalysis now underway. He might, I said, regard what was now taking place as a sort of continuation of his "first psychoanalysis" with my picture but recognize that we were now going to observe things together. My remarks relaxed him.

An exiled child

Alfonso spoke of having been put on an airplane to go to his paternal grandmother's some months after the birth of his sister, at the age of only six. He stayed with her and other relatives in Portugal for six months. He wept as he recalled crying for his mother during this time and asking for his suitcase so he could go home. I sensed that his "exile" after his sister's birth was a crucial trauma in his early life.

I now began to consider his nightly behavior with my picture as also an expression of his separation anxiety and his encouragement of his wife's (mother's) attendance at my (father's) seminar as an expression of his exile over and beyond any oedipal implications. He had repeated his childhood "exile" experience with me, giving me indirectly an idea of how he, as a child, had felt while he was in Portugal. If I were with his woman (his wife coming to my seminar), he was the rejected child. And his coming to me after one year was like an angry child's homecoming. He was always afraid of rejection, and indeed this was perhaps related to my thought of transferring him to another analyst.

When I approached the subject of his responsibility for having his wife attend my seminars, he reacted with increased intellectualization. So, I altered my technique and guided him to further disclosures about his "first psychoanalysis." I felt that differentiating me from the representation of me in his premature transference development would help prepare a foundation for the development of a more workable therapeutic alliance and transference development. As he spoke, he had some idea that he had lived his childhood exile experience during his "first psychoanalysis" and said that understanding this was important to him. We were less than two months into his psychoanalysis when he spoke of having been involved in several killings.

Killings

One Monday, Alfonso said that he felt like a murderer and suspected he had what he called a "sadistic core." He anticipated that I would find this repulsive as he muttered his confession in a new and low voice, shaking as he spoke. He told of having attended a reunion of comrades from the Vietnam War in Washington, DC, during the weekend prior to this session, and how this stirred up past events of twenty years ago, events that he had never shared with anyone.

While on patrol duty in a forest in Vietnam with another marine, Alfonso saw someone in the black pajamas of the Viet Cong, and he opened fire. It should be recalled that the Viet Cong often wore black garments. When his comrade stated that their victim had been hit in the genitals, and that he would dispatch him, Alfonso chose to do it himself. Alfonso told me that the wounded enemy knew what would happen to him. He told the wounded man, "I have to do this," though he knew that it wasn't likely the wounded man understood English. Then he shot the man and killed him.

On the following day, Alfonso told me of a second killing in the war zone. He and his comrades had opened fire on an old enemy mailman, who was walking by whistling. It was unclear whose bullet had dispatched the old man. He shouted "Mine! Mine! I opened fire first." Alfonso felt as he fired that the target was not a human being. But then he found family pictures in the dead man's wallet. One of his comrades cut a finger off the corpse and sent it to his girlfriend as a souvenir.

Alfonso then reported a third killing. He said that once he had "eye contact" with a Viet Cong nurse. He claimed that through "eye contact" a man could determine the sexual availability of a woman. After seeing the nurse with whom he had established "eye contact" in the presence of another man, an enemy, he shot them both in the back and later masturbated with thoughts of raping the nurse.

The fourth killing involved a child. While at a listening post in the countryside, Alfonso and his comrades noticed a Vietnamese child had spotted them. They caught the boy and decided that he must be killed lest he inform the Viet Cong of their presence. One soldier suggested strangling him, since this would avoid the noise of gunfire. Alfonso said in his telling of this incident, "I couldn't get into this," and the hour ended. I did not hear the rest of the story until two weeks later, when Alfonso confessed to having blown away the head of the boy as he gazed up at him with pleading eyes.

He also gave me further information about the first killing at this time. Originally, he had reported that the man he had shot was armed. But now he told me that the man was not armed and in fact might not have been a Viet Cong. Originally, Alfonso censored unpalatable facts out of his disclosures; only slowly would he speak of secret things or give me clues to them.

Hearing Alfonso's stories of these killings, so early in his psychoanalysis, rekindled in my mind the idea of whether Alfonso was analyzable. I had never been a soldier or been involved in combat. However, I was exposed to terrorism on the island of Cyprus, my birthplace, in the 1950s. When I attended medical school in Ankara, Turkey, I had a roommate who was also from Cyprus. After we had graduated, just a few months after my arrival in the United States in 1957, this fellow student was killed by the Cypriot Greek EOKA (the *Ethniki Organosis Kyprion Agoniston* or National Organization of Cypriot Fighters), inducing in me a great deal of anguish and survival guilt (Volkan, 1979). So, besides knowing that horrible things occur during wars or war-like conditions, I also sensed emotionally that people are in a different consciousness in a combat zone or during acts of terrorism.

Nevertheless, without yet knowing the full details of the meaning of the killings, I sensed that Alfonso's own psychology, his internal demands, were involved in his becoming a "killer." Also, during this time in his psychoanalysis, my connecting his killings with childhood history, his separation–individuation problems, his rage of being exiled, and his oedipal conflicts would basically stay as an intellectualized discussion between us. I felt revulsion and wondered if

I could ever evolve empathy for him. Furthermore, I thought that if his psychoanalysis made him observe and feel his personal motivations for the killings—above and beyond what being in a war dictated him to do—he would feel extreme guilt. I wondered if he could tolerate this.

How could I help him to uncover things that would make him face intolerable thoughts and sensations? Even as an already experienced psychoanalyst, I was torn internally as to what to do with this analysand. I consulted with a colleague who understood my dilemma; he left the decision about working with Alfonso up to me. I decided to go on working with Alfonso while not sharing my own internal dialogues with him.

Self-punishments

Soon, Alfonso told me stories in which he had exposed himself to extreme danger in Vietnam; he or his men could easily have been killed. I had the sense he was balancing his sadistic acts by obeying an internal demand for self-punishment. The following is an example of one such story.

While in charge of a platoon, Alfonso had seen through his binoculars a Vietnamese woman bathing. This sight aroused him sexually. When the woman hung a man's black shirt out to dry, Alfonso saw this as evidence that she had a Viet Cong lover and resolved to interfere even though he knew how dangerous such action would be for himself and his men and that it would go against his orders. With rape in mind, he ordered his men toward the girl's hut "for sexual gratification, not mere terrorism." They saw the woman was a young pubertal girl. Before the men could assault the girl, the platoon was attacked by Viet Cong in an open field they were crossing to get to the hut and was forced to retreat, very narrowly missing being totally wiped out.

It was after telling this story, with great agony, that Alfonso informed me how his whole platoon was later killed, as I had reported earlier. In reporting this, he had an abreaction on the couch: sobbing, hiding his face, and assuming the fetal position. I told him to take his time. At last, he blew his nose and commented on how bizarre it was to be emotional. At this point in his psychoanalysis, Alfonso would abruptly stop being emotional and get into an intellectualized discussion as if he would lock up his troubled self in a room in his mind.

During the next eight sessions, without my encouragement, Alfonso began giving associations to the killing incidents; we were still in the second month of his actual psychoanalysis. I had the impression that during his "first psychoanalysis" with my picture, he began going over these terrible events and that because of that he would now, so early in his actual psychoanalysis, pull out associations with intense emotions whenever he would not use encapsulation. On the surface, these associations had an oedipal theme: wanting to have a woman sexually who represents the mother and punishment by his internalized or externalized father images. This in turn would make Alfonso filled with rage against his competitor, the father, and fear retaliation by him.

His accounts of killings were accompanied by stories of having fought with other men in boot camp and overseas. He always called his opponent a "motherfucker" and while on the couch, he would scream "fucker, motherfucker, kill him!" While making associations to his killings, he would fantasize about a robber entering his house and molesting his three-year-old son, with whom he obviously associated himself. In his fantasy, he would catch the robber and torture him, holding a burning cigarette to his skin, beating, and knifing him. "I feel this terrible rage," he said, shaking.

He spontaneously connected his shooting of the Viet Cong nurse with his conscious memory of a "primal scene" episode, his sight of sexual activity between his parents, as observed or fantasized. He explained, "I would hear the mattress sounds as a child and know that my parents were having sex; my mother so beautiful, so clean, and my father with his dirty fingers, stained teeth, touching her and kissing her." Then, he reported stealing his father's condoms, as mentioned earlier.

While engaged in killing in Vietnam, he had a feeling of trying to "find someone" and had a vague awareness of trying to find his father in enemy groups to kill him. At the same time, he began to respect the Viet Cong as if he were trying to "identify with the aggressor" (A. Freud, 1936). In an attempt to escape from his Oedipus complex, while in Vietnam he also became obsessed with the idea of defecting. He stopped writing to his mother and found to his surprise that he was having warm feelings for his father. This memory was connected with a recollection that his father had expressed the fear of his son having been a "sissy" as a little boy. Alfonso thought his father would now be proud of him and his history of being a fearless warrior.

As Alfonso spoke of the Vietnam killings, other acts of aggression, the association to the primal scene, and what on the surface seemed to be oedipal material, I was always aware of the preexistent transference accomplished during his "first psychoanalysis" with my picture, his difficulty with repression (especially in relation to his mother as an object of his incestuous desires), his quick and rather open connection of his Vietnam experience with oedipal issues, his avoidance at having an observing ego work with mine, and his extreme intellectualization, encapsulation, and ritualization punctuated by outbursts. Wanting to avoid premature interpretation, I focused on the evolution of a therapeutic alliance that would contain his flooded expressions and begin to make him curious. I wanted to stimulate his observing ego and the development of a workable transference.

I concluded that he was sicker than I had thought: the killings in Vietnam, besides the realities of a war, had been associated with intrapsychic demands, the war being fortuitously an opportunity for murderous behavior. I wondered to myself if he were a fully developed sexual sadist. He had sexual discharges associated with aggressive acts and fantasies. I gathered that what he called his "sadistic core" had existed long before he became a soldier. He would give emotional accounts of evidence of this "sadistic core," only to speak on the following day in a manner that pictured him as a sophisticated intellectual.

Alfonso's wife's pregnancy

At the end of the second month of our working together, Alfonso reported that his wife was pregnant. It interested me, of course, why making his wife pregnant coincided with the start of his actual psychoanalysis. Many possibilities came to my mind. But I decided to wait and see what he would bring to his psychoanalysis.

As I will illustrate below, soon I learned that two issues were prominent among psychological factors concerning his role of making his wife pregnant. First, his mother's difficult pregnancy and delivery, and second, his mother's giving birth to his sister. Both were traumatic episodes and referred to Alfonso's attempts to separate this self-representation from the representation of his mother. Both issues also were hidden under his open oedipal preoccupations. I concluded that by making his wife pregnant, Alfonso was recalling two quite interrelated traumas from his past.

When he told me that his wife was pregnant, I said nothing to Alfonso. As I listened to him, I sensed that his main concern was the fate of the fetus: his wife could have an abortion and kill the fetus. In fact, he and she spent hours discussing the pros and cons of an abortion. It was during this time that I learned how Alfonso's mother had fallen when she was pregnant with her son and in consequence was bedridden for some months. I also learned about the difficult delivery with forceps and the mother's urinary infection.

I began to understand that the infant Alfonso had had a "first" psychological exile from his ailing and perhaps depressed postpartum mother. I thought of the possibility that his mother later responded to the very early interference in the mother–newborn relationship with a pathological reaction formation. In other words, she would not allow Alfonso to have a natural symbiotic phase and later a natural separation–individuation process. I began to think that Alfonso's mother saw him as an extension of her own body, and in turn, he developed an unconscious fantasy that his mother wanted to possess his penis.

On the couch, Alfonso was giving me information about his mother's behavior that could be interpreted as her wishing to have his penis. For example, he told me about the following incident when he was a teenager. While he was getting ready to masturbate, his mother entered his bedroom as he hastily drew a sheet over his body. When she stripped back the sheet that wrapped his naked body, both were conscious of a mutual sexual interest; this was the closest they ever came to sexual engagement. It seemed to me that he had fled his parents' home for his married lover, less from fear of punishment at the hands of his father than from fear of actual incest and his mother "possessing" his penis.

In the following free associations, I could also hear how Alfonso was torn between submitting to his mother (becoming her extension) and his rage against such a possibility. Alfonso's pregnant wife had two close female friends with whom she spent time praising Alfonso for his professional success and his intellect. When the women visited Alfonso and his wife, Alfonso sat beside them in a child-sized chair. He, by his action, "became" a child. He would suddenly grow angry and scornful toward these women.

Alfonso's wife began to bleed at the end of her fourth month of pregnancy and feared a miscarriage. Alfonso became aware of his death wish for the unborn child, who would be the second child in his family and who now symbolically stood for the second child in his parental home, his sister. Alfonso had uncensored thoughts of wanting to puncture his wife's belly. I reminded him of his "exile" when his sister was born. I suggested that his sister's birth was very traumatic for him. And he regressed on the couch and began speaking in Portuguese, identifying with the mother who had spoken to him lovingly before becoming pregnant, but also recalling the Portuguese spoken to him when he was in Portugal, in exile, and when he did not fully understand what the people were telling him.

Reaching up

Alfonso had been possessed and loved by his mother and then abandoned and exiled when she had another baby. I silently made the formulation that he was at the late oedipal age when he was sent into exile. And in his mind, this regressively reactivated the memory traces of his "first exile." On his return from Portugal, he held on to oedipal issues and remained angry toward his father and recreated an idealized mother to make her "too good to reject" him again. I was reminded of a concept, "reaching up," that was first described by Bryce Boyer (1983, 1999) as a defense mechanism. "Reaching up" refers to a patient's excessive preoccupation with a conflict and its defenses and repetitions. It is associated with a particular level of childhood development that aims to escape a more anxiety-provoking conflict belonging to a lower-level childhood development. For example, a patient's constant and sometimes dramatic preoccupation with oedipal issues can be in the service of covering up a more hurtful pre-oedipal issue. Alfonso's basic conflicts were pre-oedipal and related to his separation–individuation issues and not having a cohesive identity. His "reaching up" to oedipal issues was a defense against pre-oedipal conflicts. However, his anger toward his mother had surfaced from time to time, such as when he shot his rifle at her.

I digress here for a while to state something I learned during the second year of Alfonso's psychoanalysis that gives further insight about the link between his oedipal and pre-oedipal struggles. In his second year of analysis, Alfonso wanted to know what had actually happened to him after his sister's birth. He went to see his mother and they talked. This allowed him to establish his history more realistically. It seemed that just before the birth of his sister, Alfonso had a throat infection that required a tonsillectomy that proved to be traumatic. His mother, with the new baby, thought of him as ailing, and she had sent him to his relatives in Portugal in hopes of improving his health. The tonsillectomy was not the only body invasion the child underwent. A few months before his tonsils were removed, she consulted a physician over a swelling in his testicles. Then this physician injected the child's testicles with some medication, using a needle.

When Alfonso came back from Portugal, his mother noticed his tan and evident weight gain and no longer thought of him as damaged or ill, and the two resumed their special bond. But the effects of the exile and its link to the first "exile" remained behind the resumed bond that he needed to hold on to with open incestuous wishes and activities to try to repress the image of a rejecting mother. The interpretation of my understanding of his deep difficulties could not be made in the first year of Alfonso's psychoanalysis; this would be premature. Most likely, he would respond to it by intellectualization. I was still waiting for a full development of his "working ego" (Olinick, 1980) and for our therapeutic alliance to develop.

I will now go back to speak about what evolved next between us. When I suggested that his wife's second pregnancy might remind him of his mother's pregnancy with his sister, Alfonso pulled out more memories of staying in exile in Portugal. The flight from the United States to Portugal had been turbulent and the passengers had been anxious. One woman said her Rosary, and little Alfonso expected to die. This validated his notion that separating from his mother was like dying and that separation kills.

If Alfonso went along with my exploration of his psychological link between the present and the past for a day or two, he would soon change into a man without any psychological insight at all. He would see me as alarming and would come in "uniform," wearing a military cap, armed against me, as it were. His military cap had the legend: "Swift, silent, deadly" on it. And he would wave at me like a fly—keeping me at a distance. During these instances, he would see me as the oedipal father who was ready to kill him and who had made "my" woman (i.e., Alfonso's mother) pregnant.

Vietnam experiences

When we were in the ninth month of his actual analysis, Alfonso returned to his Vietnam experiences and began dreaming of shooting in the bush and the Viet Cong mailman he had killed. I suggested that the mailman with his pouch symbolized Alfonso's mother, who had difficulty delivering him. But I felt that I had to be careful not to make him filled with extreme guilt for the killing, and therefore I also mentioned to him about the reality of his being in a war zone, in a different consciousness, where the killing of the enemy was required. He began more openly expressing the death wish concerning his unborn child. I sensed he found it difficult to differentiate his wife's pregnancy from the second pregnancy of his mother. I offered to help him sort out the realistic problems concerning his wife's pregnancy from the things left over from the past—this soothed him, but he began to cry and shake, saying, "I can't be away from my mommy."

Full moon

Alfonso became obsessed with being an advocate for his son, whom he anticipated would feel rejected when the new baby arrived. Although the unborn baby's sex had not been ascertained, he insisted on speaking of "she" after her sister. He dreamed of having sex with someone with gray hair (a condensation of his mother and his psychoanalyst). When he inserted his penis, it went through her body as through it were a blade. He knew he was hurting her. He recalled the moans of the woman with whom he had had sex. Although she had obviously been expressing pleasure, he was frightened at the thought that he was injuring her.

About a month before his wife was expected to deliver, he became obsessed with the idea of a full moon making a werewolf or a lunatic of him. I reminded him of the belief that babies often come with a full moon. He began screaming "I don't want another child! A child will interfere with my work."

He found it hard to leave his son at nursery school and say good-bye to him. I helped him see that the boy represented himself as a small boy, deprived of his mother. I noted he was making himself a mother devoted to her son. All this drama about the child was split away from his calm, intellectualized, and seemingly sophisticated professional life. He said that after the baby came he would take a long vacation from psychoanalysis. I said that would repeat his early exiles and that there would be no vacation. "Should someone be rejected when someone else is born?" I asked him.

Returning to Vietnam experiences

Suddenly the local newspapers and television were full of accounts of a murder in the city where Alfonso and his family lived. A male student at the college where Alfonso was teaching had killed the parents of his girlfriend, stabbing them so many times that the mother was almost decapitated. Alfonso did not know this student. Between his sessions, he exhausted himself striking a punching bag. During his therapy hour, he was flooded with emotions over killings in Vietnam.

I said, "Look, news of the murder of someone's parents is making you feel guilty for crimes you did not commit; you did not actually kill your mother and sister. Your killings in Vietnam occurred when you were at war. I will continue to be curious about your internal world. But I want to continue considering that the killings took place when you were in an entirely different state of consciousness." I was offering myself to him as a less punishing and benign object. I decided to confide that also I have never been in a combat zone but I had some experience with hostility and terrorism and that I would try to understand how it must have been in Vietnam.

My remarks put a stop to his emotional flooding, and he said he feared for his son's safety. I sensed that his son again represented himself as a child. He wanted a 45-caliber pistol to protect the boy from any "intruder." I told him directly not to buy a gun but to put his thoughts and feelings into words instead.

The birth of Alfonso's daughter

Within a few days, his wife delivered a baby girl, and Alfonso gave a cool intellectual account of having been present at the delivery. The obstetrician had handed him scissors with which to cut the cord and jokingly stated, "Be careful, you wouldn't want to lose a foot." Although Alfonso was aware of not wanting this baby, and not wanting to cut the cord, he did so—taking great care not to hurt his child. He worried over whether the infant would breathe or not. That night, he had a dream in which a well-known film actress cuddled him. This same actress, however, had also been in a movie in which she mutilated people. This represented Alfonso's wish that his daughter (sister) be mutilated also.

When he asked his son if they should send the baby back, the boy said, "No Dad, I like her." The child did not accept his father's externalizations. Alfonso said that he "should have had the courtesy" to send news of the baby's birth to his sister. He did not do so. He recalled the calamity of the birth of his sister, which had caused him to be exiled to Portugal as a child. Once more, memories of the plane ride and his frantic hunt for his suitcase became very real to him and he cried out, "I'm a good boy. I want my mommy."

Again, Alfonso came to his sessions in an outfit that resembled a uniform, declaring it was time for his father to die. He dreamt of my having anal sex with him. He was paralyzed while on the couch and feared to speak lest he may say something that would "set me off." I repeated that his daughter's birth had reawakened his memory of being exiled to Portugal and that he had tried to idealize his mother when he came back from Portugal to suppress the horror of the exile. I said he could maintain this maneuver by making a scapegoat out of his father, who had never physically abused him. I told him now he was experiencing me like the father of his childhood.

I explained that Alfonso was himself creating the notion of his father's evil and that his way of dealing with trauma, however creative it might be, was not working well. All his life he had been on guard against danger from his father and mother and was wasting energy trying in a lonely way to protect himself. I asked if he would let me observe his dilemma at his side. He seemed to take this in and relaxed on the couch.

A dream about a weasel and the turning point in the treatment

At his next session, Alfonso exhibited no paralysis on the couch, nor did he experience me any longer as someone who would send him into exile. "I was creating my childhood in adult life, and how I was immersed in it. I said to myself 'Damn!' I'm calmer now but I have low-key depression. I had a weird dream." As I listened to his dream, I noticed his observing ego joining mine. His reporting this dream and his associations to it marked the turning point of his psychoanalysis.

Alfonso stated that in the dream he was in a pigpen: "Huge pigs. I was there too. But the pigs were bigger than I. At first, it did not seem to be dangerous. Suddenly one of them, a dark one, got up on his hind legs, pushed me, bit me on the shoulder."

At this point in his narrative, he touched his shoulder. It should be recalled that once in reality he had hurt his neck and shoulder after diving into shallow water in a masochistic gesture at having broken a long period of celibacy through a sexual encounter. Continuing with the story, he said, "I said to myself, 'Hey! This pig is dangerous.' I got away from him, but there was no way to get out of the pigpen. Another pig, a light one, was lying down, but I knew she was also potentially dangerous. Then I saw this weasel and knew it was dangerous, too, and that I had to protect myself from it. I found a chair and used it the way lion tamers do in the circus against the attack from the weasel. Boy, what a situation! I woke up."

Alfonso told me that when he was ten years old, he went back to Portugal with his mother for a short visit. They visited someone who had huge pigs in a cage. He was told they were dangerous, and he felt frightened. He continued, "This is the same feeling I have had in your office. Remember that I dove into shallow water and broke my neck? But the first time I dove into shallow water and hurt myself it was in Portugal, during my return when I was ten. These two pigs in my dream, one was mean and dark, and the other was female and light. My father has dark skin, and my mother's skin is light. The male pig bit me, but I had to be careful of the female pig too. I said to myself, 'Be aware of her!' The pigpen was like a gladiator's arena. One must fight to the death! Samurai! And, what about this weasel? A weasel gets its needs met. It is dangerous, very, very dangerous, tricky and sneaky and untrustworthy."

I said, "I wonder, who is this weasel? In the dream, you see your parents as dangerous. Could you consider that you are the weasel in order to protect yourself? But you don't like the weasel, you want to fight it. And this leads to a fight with yourself!"

He replied, "The weasel had a porcupine skin—sticks! Not to be beaten. There was a National Geographic show about weasels last night on the television [day residue]. Of course, those on the television were smaller than the one in my dream. But they were attacking a wolverine. Weasels are most vicious. Yes, it is disturbing to consider myself as sneaky and untrustworthy. But I must do whatever is necessary to survive. People sometimes say I am a survivor. It is a variation on my telling others, 'Give me your best shot.'"

I replied, "It seems to me that the weasel needed to be born in you for protection. But note that in your dream you are aware of an inner struggle: you are fighting the weasel, and you fight with yourself."

Alfonso went on: "I did not want to tell you this dream, but I figured out that it is important. There is more to the dream. The fence around the pigpen was wooden. I began to climb over it, but it broke down, and I was afraid that I was damaging something. I was afraid of being harmful. So, I put the fence back and got stuck in the pigpen. The fence was like a wall."

For the next month or so, Alfonso, for practical purposes, continued to give associations to this dream. He came to feel that all aspects of his conflicts belonged to him. He was the weasel and he was the one who saw the weasel as "repugnant" and fought against it. His putting a "wall" around the pigpen most likely reflected his fixation; everything in the pigpen was part of him, located in his internal world.

Alfonso took responsibility for his own psychological makeup, and we began working psychoanalytically together in earnest. We developed a good therapeutic alliance. We worked three more years and he terminated his psychoanalysis successfully. No longer was he using encapsulation and experiencing the breakup of such a defense mechanism.

He also stopped unconsciously relating to others—his children, and, in his analysis, me—as images of his childhood figures. He became a comfortable and loving husband, father, and devoted teacher.

Follow-up

Two years after his psychoanalysis was terminated, Alfonso and his family moved to a city in another state far from Virginia. Now he was the head of the sociology department at a university. A former medical student of mine, now a psychiatrist, was also a teacher at the same university. This psychiatrist would call me several times each year. On a few occasions he mentioned his and his family's wonderful new neighbors, Alfonso and his family. I never told the psychiatrist that I had worked with his new neighbor and friend.

I met Alfonso only one more time, ten years after he had completed his psychoanalysis. I was invited to give a lecture at his university. After I finished my speech, I was taken to a dinner party. I was surprised to see Professor Alfonso and his wife there. We shook hands and joined others in conversations. I noted how much Professor Alfonso was respected and loved by his colleagues. When the dinner party was over, and I was leaving to go to my hotel, he approached me and again shook my hand and whispered, "Thank you."

CHAPTER 18

Two brief psychoanalytic psychotherapy cases

Another reason why we chose to tell the story of Alfonso's first fifteen months in four-times-a-week psychoanalysis in the previous chapter is to wonder about the differences between psychoanalysis and psychoanalytic psychotherapy. Alfonso's case was complicated, primarily because Alfonso's emotions related to the wartime killing of others and the loss of his own men.

Alfonso was extremely traumatized when his platoon was brutally killed and he survived. After he took care of the "weasel" within and made positive internal changes, he was able, in the third year of his psychoanalysis, to relive his Vietnam experiences on the couch.

In the transference, his analyst began to represent the Viet Cong. Alfonso began coming to his sessions dressed like a soldier. Session after session he would suddenly sit up on the couch and use an imaginary machine gun to shoot at the wall in front of him while making machine-gun sounds: "Ta ta ta ta ta." Sometimes, he would use his imaginary machine gun during almost the entire session. For over a month, Vamık Volkan had to be able to sit behind him, stay silent, and sense his rage, guilt, and fear. Since Alfonso's work during the previous years had produced an underlying trust and positive transference, he never turned his imaginary machine gun toward his psychoanalyst. Together, Alfonso and Vamık Volkan were able to observe the horror of murdering others in a war zone and the survivor guilt he had experienced. By the end of his analysis Alfonso was able to master and tolerate such disturbing psychological processes successfully and develop an identity as a good person with high-level internal organization.

We suspect that if Alfonso were seeing a psychotherapist face-to-face once or twice a week in psychoanalytic psychotherapy, he would not be able to use the imaginary machine gun that helped him to make drastic positive changes in his internal world. However, every patient we see does not have as complicated an internal world as Alfonso had prior to his psychoanalysis. Our experiences indicate that successful long-term psychoanalytic psychotherapies that remove the patient's pathological symptoms and help the patient to deal with issues that had brought him or her to treatment are what many individuals seek, without needing to accomplish more generalized and sometimes drastic modifications of the patient's internal world.

There are different types of psychoanalytically informed psychotherapies. Here we present two of Vamık Volkan's brief case studies. The first is the psychotherapy of an eight-year-old boy. This case uses the technique of making psychoanalytically informed suggestions to the parents. The second case focuses on psychoanalytic findings on loss and mourning and helping a patient facing recent loss go through an uncomplicated mourning process.

An eight-year-old boy who shit his pants

My shortest psychoanalytical psychotherapy experience took place in 1960 when I was still a psychiatric resident at the University of North Carolina Hospital. This experience included a psychoanalytically informed suggestion. My patient, Oliver, was an eight-year-old boy. His symptom was defecating into his pants whenever he left his elementary school and came close to entering his family house. This behavior had continued for four months when his mother brought him for outpatient treatment. I was assigned to treat Oliver. When I interviewed him, Oliver had no insight into his symptom. Since he seemed to be embarrassed, I did not push him to tell me things that he was hesitant to reveal.

When I interviewed Oliver's mother, she told me that her husband was away from the United States for about two years as part of his military service. During this time, she felt very lonely in the family's home. This led her to sleep with her son every night. She and Oliver were informed that Oliver's father was going to return home; but they did not know the exact day and time of his arrival. When the father entered the family house, instead of hugging his wife and son, he shouted at Oliver's mother and said, "When I was away who were you sleeping with?" The boy witnessed this scene.

That evening, Oliver began to sleep again in his own bed in a room next to the parental bedroom, and most likely heard the very loud arguments taking place in the parental bedroom. Oliver's mother told me that she did not have a love affair when her husband was away. But her husband's suspicions continued as did arguments and verbal fights between him and her. She then refused to share a bed with him, and her husband began to sleep with her son. Her son's symptom of defecating into his pants started about two months after the son and father began sharing a bed. Oliver's mother had no connection in her mind between her son's symptom and the story she told me. As a young, psychoanalytically informed therapist, I immediately thought that the story I heard had inflamed oedipal issues in the boy. The boy's symptom represented a need to keep his father away who, in the boy's unconscious fantasy, not only could castrate his son but also could molest him while lying next to him in the same bed. If he used an anal defense mechanism—feces in his pants—he would keep the dangerous father away.

Using my psychoanalytic understanding of their son's symptom, I met with Oliver's mother and father. Without using any technical terms, I explained to them my understanding of their son's problem. I also created a situation during which Oliver's mother re-confirmed that she had always been a faithful wife and that she really wanted to be loved by her husband. I also firmly told the parents that from that day forward Oliver should sleep alone in his bed. I met with Oliver and informed him what I had suggested to his parents without making an interpretation, Instead, I mentioned that the parents will sleep together and that when he sleeps in his own bed alone, he will have a sense of his own freedom. The parents did what I told them right away. The husband and wife began to sleep together again. Meanwhile, I saw Oliver once a week for about five months. We played games of soldiers and I learned more about the boy's fantasies about his soldier father when he was away. He volunteered to tell me how, in his mind, he would try to measure the distances, sometime a few inches, between his body and his father's body while they were in the same bed. I indirectly encouraged him, and also his father, to play ball together on the weekends. Also, the reader should know that a few weeks after Oliver's father stopped sleeping with him, Oliver's symptom had disappeared.

Oliver and his mother came to see me six months after I stopped working with Oliver. I learned that Oliver's symptom never returned. Oliver's mother agreed to call me after another six months passed. When she did, she reported that everyone in the family was living comfortably, and that she and her husband were planning to have a second baby.

The case of a red robe

Julia, a single African American woman in her mid-thirties, functioned well as a secretary at a local business office. Six months after her mother's death, however, she was unable to carry on her secretarial work. Her employer demanded that she get help in order to keep her job. I saw her face-to-face daily, except for the weekends. Her treatment took place over only one and a half months.

Julia was the youngest of six children in her family. Her mother had been severely burned when Julia was six months old. Bedridden for a year, the mother had been unable to carry out many of her mothering functions, but there were mother substitutes: older sisters and some relatives. Nevertheless, the early mother–daughter relationship contained elements of unresolved separation–individuation conflicts, manifested in later years as sadomasochism.

Although her siblings all left home, Julia stayed with her widowed mother in the last ten years of her life, when her mother became an amputee because of diabetes. Since Julia's mother spent most of her time in bed or seated in an armchair, Julia brought her food, cleaned her, and literally became her maid. Julia had surrendered all independent social life, a college scholarship, and opportunities for marriage to care for her mother. The family did not have money to hire someone to look after Julia's mother.

Although Julia sometimes was conscious of a wish for her mother's death, she kept in touch with her night and day at regular intervals "to see if she was all right." Julia phoned her mother several times a day from the place where she worked as a secretary, and slept at the foot of her bed, checking her mother's state periodically during the night.

A little over six months after her mother's death, Julia was flooded with different images of her mother, to which she related with ambivalence. Dreams of "saving" and "getting rid of" her mother awakened Julia with anxiety each night, and she suffered from loss of sleep. By day, she was so greatly occupied with her mother's images that she was unable to carry out her secretarial work and was in danger in losing her job. Julia complained that her mother was driving her crazy.

A typical adult-type response to meaningful loss includes grief reaction and the work of mourning. If the mourner is not prepared to face the loss, the grief reaction includes shock, denial, and bargaining to reverse the outcome, pain, and anger, all of which—especially anger—eventually lead to the beginning of an emotional "knowledge" that the lost object is indeed gone. Before grief is completed, the work of mourning begins. Mourning refers to revisiting, reviewing, and transforming the mourner's emotional investment in the images of the lost object. It comes to a practical end when such preoccupations, with associated affects, lose their intensity.

During the diagnostic interview, I made a case formulation that Julia was unable to get on with her work due to complications in grieving and mourning. In my formulation, I noted that Julia needed to keep her dead mother alive in order to make her "good" by her own efforts and attention. Once her mother had become "good," Julia could achieve psychological freedom from her or separate from her without guilt. This wish to "save" her mother conflicted with her wish to "get rid of" the woman to whom she had served as a chronic caretaker. At the time of the older woman's death, Julia had also disruptively identified with her mother's mental representation.

The diagnostic interview revealed the existence of a special object, a red robe that Julia said had belonged to both her and her mother. Several years earlier, a sibling had relieved Julia in caring for her mother, and Julia had been able to take a pleasure trip to a big city, where she had bought what she thought of as a "sexy" red robe. On her return, her mother expressed a desire for it, and Julia had given it to her. What had once symbolized her freedom from her mother now symbolized her submission to an abusing mother. The women alternated wearing this red robe. Finally, the mother's condition grew so alarming that an ambulance had been called; she wanted to wear the red robe on her trip to the hospital, and indeed, was wearing it in the hospital when she died.

After the funeral, Julia's siblings gathered in their mother's home and busied themselves "protecting Julia" from confronting the sad reminders of the dead woman, taking away almost all the mother's belongings. But Julia kept the red robe. She put it away in a brown grocery bag that she sealed shut and hid it in a corner of a closet. As time went on, Julia realized that it had come to have magical properties and that she was afraid to touch it. It gave her eerie spells; she had to reassure herself about its whereabouts but also distance herself from it. Julia did not have breaks from reality, except for certain fantasies and visual hallucinations in which she seemed to see different images of her mother in the air, and dreams in which her mother appeared in the red robe.

I told Julia that she had complications in her mourning process and that during our meetings, we would try to make sense of her chaotic memories, fantasies, dreams, and hallucinations. Julia's hallucinations decreased considerably during the first week of her treatment. Instead, she felt very disturbed by her dreams, which she said were "killing" her. In one dream, her mother lay in a coffin but was attempting to get out. Julia then called the undertaker to give her mother "a shot of something to calm her down."

From the start of her psychotherapy, I tried to use the manifest content of her dreams to show her that she was engaged in a struggle to decide whether to rescue her mother or let her die. The goal here was to clarify the complications that obstructed her mourning and to help her deal with them; no deeper understanding of her dreams was attempted. I collected data about Julia's relationship with her mother from childhood and attempted to develop a therapeutic alliance with her by suggesting that all the "bizarre" dreams, fantasies, and hallucinations would start being less bothersome for her once her mourning got on the right track.

I asked Julia to bring a picture of her mother, and she did, during the fifth hour, although she refused to look at it until later. After three more sessions were concluded, she looked at it, screaming, "That's her!" and then started crying. She refused to face the picture while she cried, since "mother never cried, not even when daddy died." I learned that Julia's father had died some ten years previously.

The next three sessions saw the outpouring of more memories. Julia's preoccupation with her mother changed from the reality of her abuse at her mother's hands to transient sadness about her death. She was able to verbalize having wished from time to time that her mother was dead. To indicate my acceptance of her conflicting views of her mother, I told Julia that from what she had told me she had good reasons for her opposing perceptions of her mother.

I then asked Julia to bring the red robe to therapy because I thought that looking and touching this special object might help her put her feelings and thoughts about her mother into words. The next day, she brought the red robe in its paper bag and put it on the floor in my office. She postponed touching the bag and then started screaming, "Let me out of here! I can't stand it!" She was referring to her wish to run away from the powerful vindictive parent. During later sessions in which she was asked to touch and examine the robe, to describe it, and feel free to verbalize all of the feelings it evoked, Julia was flooded with emotions of anger and sadness, and wept, giving more details about the day of her mother's death.

I learned that when she had gone forward to look at her mother's corpse, Julia had fainted, and, as a result, had never seen the corpse. She had left the cemetery before the coffin was lowered into the ground. I told her that these circumstances supported her attempt to deny that her mother was dead. She discussed the funeral in detail and recalled the sermon the minister had preached during the service. She confessed how she had wanted praise at the funeral and how the minister had applauded her masochistic devotion and wished her luck and happiness in her new freedom. Since she was at the time fully aware of her anger toward her mother, these remarks had evoked intense feelings of guilt.

Julia brought a dream that her mother was in a casket. She said: "The casket is small now, like a box. My mother is also small. She is shrunken!" I told her that her unresolved guilt was keeping her mother "big" and that, with the lessening of her guilt, her mother would shrink further.

Almost after a month since we started to work together, Julia dreamed of a cemetery in which mourners, her mother among them, looked disappointed at the absence of a grave. "I was able to look in my dream at the site where my mother was buried," Julia said. "But there was no grave; the ground was all covered by grass!" This dream had been followed on the same night by one in which I performed "eye surgery" on her. Again, connecting the manifest content to her disturbed grieving and mourning process, I suggested that she was perceiving me as an "eye-opener" who would help her to see the reality of her mother's death, and that she was caught between "seeing" and "not seeing"—keeping "alive" or keeping "dead"—her mother. In a third dream on the same night, Julia saw a nurse erase an image of her mother that had been drawn on a blackboard.

On the next evening, Julia dreamed of seeing her mother. "This time she looked like a ghost and she could go in and out of a wall. In the dream, she retreated into a wall." Julia talked further about the funeral and expressed more anger about the minister's praise of her masochistic behavior. The next evening, she dreamed of her mother in a wheelchair; Julia pushed the wheelchair off a cliff and noticed that her mother did not seem to object. After reporting this dream, she talked about the funeral, with tears in her eyes.

Julia then dreamed of her mother sitting on the porch of their home. She said to her mother, "You are dead," and when the older woman refused to believe her, Julia called a mortician, who carried her mother away in a casket. After Julia had this dream, the photograph and the red robe, which had been left in my office and continued to be available to her whenever she had a session, now seemed to lose their magic. She asked if she could have them back, and when I offered no objection, she took them away with her.

Julia told me that she had been looking at advertisements for tombstones. Although she had arranged for a marker to be placed on her father's grave within a month after his death, she had been unable, eight months after her mother's death, to order one for her. She could now talk more realistically than before about the death and was no longer intensively preoccupied with thoughts of her mother.

Two sessions later, Julia announced that she had burned the red robe and ordered a tombstone. Then I received more history of her mother's being burned and having been made unavailable to give her adequate mothering during her childhood. Now, I realized that she was symbolically trying to get rid of the "burned mother" image. Julia elaborated further, with emotions, on the remembered problems of being a child of a burned woman.

Julia had been afraid to return to the cemetery since the burial, and was anxious at first over a proposed visit, the possibility of which was raised in her psychotherapy. She doubted that she would be able to go through with it. Then she brought a dream of being at her mother's grave. She said: "I was able to see the grave this time, and there was a marker on it, but I kept digging into it. I wanted to reach my mother to give her flowers, but I never reached her." Julia wept aloud while reporting this dream and displayed genuine sadness.

The next day, without my suggestion, she took a weekend trip as a tourist to the city where she had bought the red robe. There, she had a "wonderful time." She reported being proud of herself and of being able to go through grieving. A couple of days later, she dreamed of buying new shoes. Her associations were to visiting the big city and having fun doing so. Then Julia visited her mother's grave, and her psychotherapy that had focused on the complications of her grieving and mourning processes came to an end.

Follow-up

Julia was one of the individuals who had agreed to participate in a follow-up study of patients after receiving psychotherapy for complicated mourning, which Vamık Volkan named "re-grief therapy" (V. D. Volkan, 1981). In the first letter, written a year after her treatment ended, Julia reported working and "feeling simply wonderful." She added: "I am no longer afraid of the dark, of being alone, of expressing my true feelings." Her last letter, written three years after her treatment ended, also gave testimony to her well-being. At that time, Julia was planning to move to a new location and she wrote, "As a matter of fact, everything is going fine for me these days."

CHAPTER 19

A psychotherapy case with cultural considerations

The following case is about a woman who was seen by Kevin Volkan in a community counseling center in a poor neighborhood in Los Angeles. In many aspects, this case is a typical representation of psychoanalytic psychotherapy. However, the cultural background of the patient played an important role in the patient's treatment. This serves to remind us that patients' cultural backgrounds influence their lives in important ways, and this needs to be examined in psychotherapy.

Case example of Isabella

Isabella, a Latina woman in her early thirties, was referred to me by the California Victims Witness program that assists victims of crime to obtain psychotherapy and other services. She was referred for psychotherapy after being beaten by her husband. A few days after this beating had occurred, Isabella's social worker observed Isabella becoming agitated while mumbling to herself in English and Spanish, throwing things around her home, crying out, and acting dissociated. I saw Isabella in a community counseling center located in a barrio in southern California. This was a very rough neighborhood, with high rates of violence, drug addiction, and gang warfare. An experience I had on my first day of working at this counseling center will illustrate the nature of the neighborhood. As I was driving to the counseling center and about a block from turning into the building, I looked out of my car window and saw a man lying on his back on the front lawn of his house. Sticking up from his body was a large butcher's knife plunged about halfway into his chest. As I drove by, I could hear sirens. Within seconds, police cars and paramedics had driven on to the lawn, and first responders swarmed over the scene, working to stabilize the victim.

Isabella had grown up in the barrio and lived there most of her life. Besides her parents, she was raised with two older brothers. The two brothers had become successful enough to move out of the barrio, leaving Isabella to take care of her parents. Isabella's father had worked in a factory that processed asbestos most of his career. He now suffered from asbestosis, a condition where exposure to asbestos over the years causes scarring and thickening of the lung tissue. He had also smoked for many years. Isabella reported that he was slowly dying from this condition.

While Isabella was growing up, her mother worked odd jobs—such as cleaning and doing laundry—and functioned as a traditional housewife running the household. In their youth, both parents had come from Mexico to the United States as farm workers picking vegetables and strawberries. Both parents had received no more than an elementary school education. Neither spoke English or Spanish well, and the Mixtec language was used at home. Both parents were devout Catholics.

Isabella reported that her father was very stern and had used corporal punishment on his children—typically a spanking or sometimes a switch. Isabella reported that her father had been affectionate toward her when she was young, holding her and giving her hugs and kisses. However, after her *quinceañera* (coming-of-age party) on her fifteenth birthday, he became aloof and distant and no longer gave her any physical contact. Nevertheless, he asserted a good deal of control over Isabella's life, even after she was an adult. Isabella's mother was unassertive and devoted herself to taking care of her children and husband, as well as being involved with her church. My impression of Isabella's mother from Isabella's description was that she was depressed. Isabella reported that her father had been violent toward her mother in the past, but he was too physically frail to hit anyone now.

Isabella had not received any education about birth control growing up and had become pregnant at twenty after one of her first sexual encounters. Her father tracked down the boy who had gotten Isabella pregnant and forced him to marry Isabella, who subsequently gave birth to a boy. A few years later, Isabella had another child with her husband, this time a girl. Isabella's husband had become involved with a gang and sold drugs. Eventually, he started using his own product and became a heroin addict. Because of his addiction, he would skim heroin from the supply given to him by the gang and dilute it before it was sold. After the gang leaders became aware of this, Isabella's husband's status in the gang was greatly diminished. He was seen as unreliable and was only occasionally allowed to sell drugs for the gang. In order to support his heroin habit, he resorted to robbing houses. He would also take whatever money he could find from Isabella, who was very poor and supported her children by working as a maid in a hotel. On several occasions, Isabella's husband had taken her rent money as well as money she needed to feed her children. When Isabella would try to stop him from taking her money, he would beat her.

This had occurred right before I started working with Isabella. She continued to be assaulted for a few months after beginning psychotherapy, even though she had a restraining order against her husband. He would come to her home and beg to be let in. Isabella would relent and let him in, thereby invalidating the court order. Then the husband would again take Isabella's money and beat her. This pattern repeated itself many times in the beginning of my time working with Isabella.

When I first met Isabella, she had superficial but somewhat spectacular injuries. Half of her face and the backs of her arms were badly bruised from the beatings she had endured. One beating had been observed by a neighbor, who called the police, resulting in the husband's arrest. After the police interviewed Isabella, she was contacted by a social worker, who enrolled her in the Victim Witness program that paid her psychotherapy fees directly to the counseling center. Isabella would not otherwise have been able to afford psychotherapy, nor is it likely she would have ever sought psychotherapy on her own, since it was something, she later explained to me, that people from her neighborhood thought was only for "rich whites."

My first clinical impression of Isabella was that she had a great deal of anxiety and perhaps suffered from some dissociation. Initially, I thought she might be suffering from borderline personality disorder. However, in discussions with a more experienced colleague, I learned that people from Latino communities sometimes present symptoms in a culturally specific fashion. In Isabella's case, her presentation fit well with the culture-bound syndrome *ataques de nervios*, which is usually brought on by some sort of trauma, oftentimes related to family conflict. This syndrome can include several somatic symptoms that are related to anxiety such as heart palpitations, trembling, and pseudo-seizures. Although similar to an anxiety or panic attack, *ataques de nervios* is usually triggered by ongoing trauma and can include dissociative symptoms as well as hallucinations (Streltzer, 2017).

During Isabella's first sessions, her overriding concern was on how to keep her husband from coming over to her house. She consistently asked for advice about this. I gently told her that procuring restraining orders and interacting with the police was something her social worker would help her with, and my role was to help her understand why she was in the situation she was in. In Isabella's mind, a "counselor" (I worked out of a "counseling" center) was someone who would tell her what to do. I told Isabella that I was not going to tell her what to do but instead, help her become clear in her own mind about what she needed to improve her situation. At first, this was confusing to her.

When I brought up the question of whether she had sought help before from a counselor or doctor, Isabella told me that her mother had insisted that she see a *curandero,* a traditional folk healer, when they were in Mexico visiting family. The *curandero* she saw lived near her relatives and Isabella reported that there was always a line around the block of people waiting to see him. *Curanderos* (or *curanderas,* as they are often women) can specialize in herbal medicine, bone setting, physical manipulation of the body (akin to massage therapy, physical therapy, or chiropractic), midwifery, spiritual healing, and counseling. Nowadays, many *curanderos* also incorporate aspects of Latin American shamanism into their practices, for example, channeling of and communicating with spirit beings, manipulating energy, entering trance states, and interpreting dreams. *Curanderos* typically use more than one modality, although they may have more expertise in some than others. *Curanderos* also will use aspects of Catholicism, such as veneration and prayers to various saints, to help facilitate healing (Hendrickson, 2015).

In Isabella's case, the *curandero* performed a ritual called a *limpia*, or "cleansing." The ritual is used to remove the negative effects of a fright or trauma that the patient has experienced. Brett Hendrickson (2015) describes the *limpia* as follows:

> The basic therapies of curanderismo today generally include some talk therapy along with a limpia, a "cleansing" that removes negative and harmful energies from the body and helps restore the person to health. Starting from the crown of the head and continuing down to the feet, the curandera/o uses a small branch of herbs or an egg to sweep and rub the body clean. Traditionally, the healer prays during this ritual, making petitions on behalf of the sick and asking for divine assistance. After the limpia, the herbs or egg are destroyed so that the negative energy cannot re-infect the patient or others. A limpia also can be the first treatment in soul retrieval, needed when a person has experienced a "susto," fright or trauma that has dislocated part or all of the soul. (pp. 30–31)

The *limpia* Isabella described being performed by her *curandero* was similar to the above depiction. Isabella had undergone the *limpia* several times as well as having had spiritual healing and counseling sessions with the *curandero*. During her counseling sessions, the *curandero* had talked with Isabella about her dreams and had given her advice regarding her husband. This counseling occurred after the *curandero* had gone into a trance and was told by spirit beings that Isabella's husband was possessed by malign spirits and that she should stay away from him. Isabella was also given herbal remedies that she reported calmed her anxiety. This is not surprising since many herbal remedies made by *curanderos* are known to have psychoactive properties.

Isabella described undergoing the *limpia* as a good experience and said she always felt better afterwards. However, the good feelings would fade away after a few days, and the ritual did not solve her problems with her husband.

I felt that Isabella's experience with the *curandero* and the *limpia* were potentially positive for our sessions, with some reservations. There was a good deal of distrust of modern medicine and psychology in Isabella's family. The fact that there were similarities between psychotherapy and Isabella's experience with the *curandero* allowed her to form a therapeutic alliance with me. Entering a hypnogogic state, talking about herself, and telling her dreams would seem familiar after her traditional healing experience. On the other hand, undergoing the *limpia* was immediately cathartic and I worried that the inevitably slower process of psychotherapy would be overly frustrating. Also, the *curandero* was directive, telling Isabella to stay away from her husband. I was also worried that Isabella would have a built-in transference from her experience with the *curandero*.

I scheduled with Isabella to see her once a week since this is what the Victim Witness program would cover. Initially, the chairs in the consultation room were arranged to be face-to-face. During my first sessions with Isabella, I explained that she should say whatever came into her mind and not censor herself. She dutifully told me her recent history and about her experiences with the *curandero*. Subsequently, I arranged the chairs so that they were not facing directly toward one another, and I kept the light in the room low. I realized that my initial formulation of Isabella's personality organization as being at the borderline level was mistaken.

In our first few months together, I was able to see that Isabella's personality organization was at an oedipal level. We were quickly able to establish a therapeutic alliance, and she exhibited a positive transference toward me. It was possible that this was due to some built-in transference from the *curandero*. Isabella would at times comment how I looked like the *curandero* and he began to make appearances in her dreams as a heroic figure who would save her from unseen evil people. I initially did not comment on this. During this time, Isabella began to exhibit repetition compulsion and superego resistances. The repetition compulsion resistance was the most worrisome because it took the form of Isabella letting her husband back into her house, which would nullify the restraining order against him. Sometimes she would sleep with him, and sometimes he would beat her. After being beaten, she would call her social worker and get the restraining order reinstated.

I was lucky that the social worker usually took care of helping Isabella with the restraining orders, and I only had to do this once when the social worker was on vacation. After a few of these episodes, I made comments to Isabella to the effect that when she let her husband back into the house, our sessions were spent dealing with the consequences of this and that this perhaps took us away from getting to the root of her issues. After an episode with her husband, Isabella would come to her session with intense feelings of guilt about letting him back in the house. These sessions would be full of self-recrimination. I believed this to be a form of superego resistance. Again, I would comment to her that when she felt guilty, this kept her from making progress in therapy. Later, I combined the above interpretations and suggested to Isabella that letting her husband back in the house and then feeling guilt about it was a way she prevented herself from going deeper into therapy. This pattern of Isabella letting the husband into the house and then feeling guilty lasted about six months. One day, Isabella came to the office and proudly told me that her husband had come over and begged to be let in, but she had steadfastly refused. The husband then banged on the front door and windows, threatening her. Isabella said she had an epiphany that she was not going to let him in. She kept the door locked and called the police, who came and arrested the husband.

Isabella's resistance next took the form of transference resistance, which may have been exasperated by the built-in transference from the *curandero*. After being able to keep her husband out of her house, Isabella became discouraged with her psychotherapy. Her expectations of me were that I would magically be able to cure her like the *curandero*. But like her experience with the *curandero*, once the immediate good cathartic feeling was over, she felt somewhat depressed that more was not being accomplished. Here, the positive transference Isabella had toward me had become negative, and she voiced how she felt I had abandoned her and let her down. During this time, Isabella told me a dream:

> I was in Mexico and there was a big party. Everyone was getting presents, but somehow, no one gave me anything. There were people dancing in the streets, but half-naked, like a festival in Brazil. Everyone was happy, but I was alone and ignored. Then there was a procession, like a parade, and in the middle was the curandero; he was smiling and holding a

statue of an Aztec god. The curandero smiled at me and waved to me to come over. I became anxious and woke up.

I then asked Isabella if the *curandero* in the dream reminded her of anyone. She said, "Yes, he looks like you." I wondered to her whether the disappointment in the dream might be like the disappointment she felt in her therapy about my not being able to fix her quickly like the *curandero*. Isabella dwelt on that for a bit and then said, "Yes, it feels the same."

I then asked Isabella if the party reminded her of anything. She said that when she was younger, there had been times when her family was so poor that she and her siblings had received no Christmas presents. I asked if there were other times when there was a party and she had been disappointed. She then recalled her *quinceañera* and how happy she was initially, but then afterwards, her father wouldn't hug her anymore and seemed distant. She had felt that there was something wrong with her—that she must have done something wrong. I asked her whether her feelings of disappointment might represent what she felt when her father stopped giving her attention.

At our next session, Isabella said she wanted to talk about the dream more. I asked if there was anything in particular about the dream she was interested in. She said she realized the statue in the dream was of *Xipe Totec*—the Aztec god of fertility. As a teenager, she had seen the statue before and was shocked by it. The statue had an open mouth and a large penis, and the god was said to be wearing a cape made from flayed human skin. I asked her whether the statue might represent a manifestation of love and violence together. In the next sessions, Isabella recalled how her father used to beat her and her brothers when they were kids, but that she felt that he loved her too. I wondered out loud if perhaps she had felt that love and violence needed to be together and to get love she needed to also put up with the beatings. Isabella was able to make the connection of this to her relationship with her husband.

I believed that Isabella was making excellent progress in therapy. At a subsequent session, Isabella came in and said she was feeling anxious and guilty. I asked her to say whatever came to mind. She started crying and said she couldn't tell me. I didn't push her about this and waited.

The theme of disappointment in what she experienced as her father's rejection and the combination of love and violence filled our time. Finally, Isabella came to a session and said she had a memory:

> When I was a teenager, one of my chores was to do the laundry at home. My mother would be working, and my father would come home exhausted, grab a beer, and go outside to smoke. My father worked in a factory that made stuff from asbestos, and when he came home his clothes would be contaminated. We were told to wash his clothes separate from everyone else's. One time, I was doing the laundry and I put my father's work clothes in the washer. I was in a bad mood and feeling lazy, so I put my mom's clothes in with my dad's so I wouldn't have to do another wash. I thought no one will ever know. Just remembering this I feel so guilty, I could have made my mom sick!

During the next couple of months, Isabella talked a lot about her mother, who seemed to have been depressed much of the time and who suffered somewhat at the hands of Isabella's father, who was demanding of his wife. Isabella's mother was expected to take care of the home and the children, as well as bring in money from outside work. Isabella began to recall that there were times when the father slapped her mother when he was displeased. During this time, Isabella began to sympathize with her mother and to see how some of her own patterns of relating were similar. Isabella came in one session and declared that she was determined not to end up like her mother. She decided that she was going to go back to school so she could have a career and make enough money to take care of herself and her children.

She was also determined to move out of her old neighborhood. This occurred after about two years or 100 hours of psychotherapy. This was also just about the time when the Victim Witness program funding for Isabella's psychotherapy was finished. At this point, I felt that Isabella might benefit from group psychotherapy, and I recommended that she join a psychotherapy group. I made this recommendation for three reasons. The first was that the psychotherapy group was run by myself and a female coleader. My thought was that the experience of working with a female psychotherapist would give Isabella a chance to explore more of her feelings around her mother. The second reason was that this particular psychotherapy group consisted of career women who might serve as role models or examples for Isabella. The third reason was that group psychotherapy was inexpensive enough that Isabella would be able to afford to pay for it on her own. Isabella subsequently joined the psychotherapy group that she attended for a year. At the end of the year, Isabella was enrolled in a nursing degree program and her schedule was such that she couldn't attend the group psychotherapy sessions, so she left the group. Both the co-therapist and I felt that Isabella had made excellent progress in group psychotherapy.

CHAPTER 20

Psychoanalytic ideas related to organizations and groups

In Chapter 11, we wrote about political leaders—the pole of ethnic, national, religious, and ideological large-group tents—and described reparative and destructive ones with exaggerated narcissism. We gave examples of how sometimes clinicians will need to pay great attention to their patients' investments in such large-group identities and prejudice against the other. In Chapter 11, the term large group referred to thousands or millions of people sharing a historical background and the same sentiments. In this section, we expand upon Freud's ideas about the role of group members and leaders in smaller work and organizational groups, though much of the material here is relevant to larger groups as well. We can begin by using a simple organizational case study of Kevin Volkan's as an example.

Case example of an organization

I worked as a consultant to a medium-sized technology company in the San Francisco Bay area. There had been some tension between the engineering staff and management, and my job was to study what was going on in the company and make recommendations on how to alleviate the problems. Along with this, I provided training in conflict resolution starting with upper management and working down through the employee ranks. The vice president who had hired me made sure that all the upper management went through a communications strategy training program, himself included. This program taught non-authoritative communication techniques as well as an understanding of both conscious and unconscious factors that different types of employees used to communicate. The upper-level managers were excited about the program and eager to learn tools to increase communication and problem-solving skills in the company. After completing the program, upper management staff rated it highly and felt that it was valuable for them.

The program was then offered to mid-level managers, and the vice president showed up on the first day to give the program his official blessing. At the end of the first day, the middle managers were elated about the program and the adoption of non-authoritarian communication techniques by the company. However, when they returned to their offices at the end of the day, they found an unwanted surprise. The vice president had issued a memo stating that he would no longer tolerate employees who came to work late. All employees, even those just a few minutes late, would have their pay docked for lateness. There were to be no exceptions. Even though this scenario happened years ago, this sort of authoritarian policy is now taking the form of restriction on, or bans on, working from home in the wake of Covid-19. Elon Musk's recent missive to Tesla employees stating that he expected them in the office for a minimum of forty hours a week is a good example of this sort of thing (Musk, 2022).

After this memo was sent out, no one groaned louder than the middle managers who had spent a day immersed in non-authoritative communication techniques. The vice president's new tardiness memo seemed to contradict everything they had just been taught. The next day one of the middle managers approached me and vented her frustration. I suggested that she use some of the skills that she had just been taught to initiate a conversation about the memo with the vice president. This middle manager thought about it but decided that since the vice president had a history of making sudden and seemingly unwarranted policy changes it would be better not to confront him and face possible retribution. Soon after this, the positive feelings about the non-authoritative communication training faded away. The middle managers felt that the program was an exercise in futility and did not promote it to their employees. Nevertheless, the vice president believed that the program was a huge success and was not shy about taking credit for instituting a culture change in the organization. He seemed blissfully unaware that this change never actually occurred.

This simple example demonstrates the importance of psychological pathology in group leaders. In the case of many organizations, this pathology is subtle. The vice president in the example had said one thing but done something else. It seemed as if his need to be an authority figure undermined his desire to improve communication skills among the employees. Even a well-designed intervention could not change a maladaptive leadership style that was unconscious in origin. It is our contention that neglect of unconscious forces acting in groups and group leaders is often responsible for the failure of interventions to inspire positive changes in organizations. Understanding of these unconscious aspects is a key element in understanding group behavior.

Psychoanalytic understanding of groups

Freud believed that for the most part, individual psychology was bound to the psychology of the group, and group psychology consisted of the psychology of the individuals making up a group (Freud, 1921c). Another way of understanding this is to state that group identification is a necessary component of the human mind.

Humans naturally form groups. Primates form groups because group membership has survival value, which is also true for human groups. The size of primate groups is related to the ability to recognize group members. This limits the size of nonhuman primate groups since recognition is primarily through grooming, which is a time-intensive task. Humans can recognize group membership through use of language, which has allowed humans to form much larger social groups. Human groups are limited by the ability to cooperate and to detect "cheaters"— individuals who do not contribute to the group but take advantage of the cooperative behavior of others (Czárán & Aanen, 2016; Dunbar, 1993). In psychoanalytic theory, naturally forming groups are understood as having a "collective mind" that differs from the mind of the individual. The conscious mind of the individual is lost in this type of group and is replaced by the largely unconscious group mind. For this unconscious group mind to exist, there must be something that holds the group together. This is accomplished through the unconscious identification of the group members with each other and the group leader. This process of identification reduces the rational processes of the group members and increases their emotions. The process of becoming a group member begins when an individual yields to his or her unconscious instincts and joins a group. The unconscious instincts (id) of the individual are now able to overcome repression (by the ego) because the power of the group supports the expression of unconscious wishes. Every sentiment and emotion becomes highly contagious in a group, causing individuals to sacrifice their personal interests to accomplish the group task. For "normal" functioning human groups, this can be understood as a form of sublimation.

Emotions in a group are overwhelming and hypnotic in power, and the individual loses his or her conscious personality and independent will, both of which are replaced to some extent with the personality and will of the group. This mutual identification brings with it a sense of purpose as well as a loss of self. Because of these qualities, groups are simultaneously capable of realizing high ideals and committing all manner of atrocities. Indeed, the contradictory nature of groups, fueled by their unconscious goals, often causes them to be out of sync with reality. As Freud (1921c) wrote:

> And finally, groups have never thirsted after truth. They demand illusions, and cannot do without them. They constantly give what is unreal precedence over what is real; they are almost as strongly influenced by what is untrue as by what is true. (p. 80)

In Freud's work *Totem and Taboo* (1912–13), he characterizes the group leader as a primal father. This primal father is killed by an alliance of sons, and his rule is replaced by totemic law. This prevents rivalry and incest among the group members. Freud's metaphor mirrors modern research on the formation of early human groups. At some point, groups evolved to such a size and complexity that detection of cheating became difficult without formalized rules for group members (Czárán & Aanen, 2016). Once these rules were established and codified into language, human groups could become larger, and the group tasks more compli-cated. For Freud, this led to the development of civilization. This devel-opment required, however, that group members sublimated their sexual and aggressive urges to an even greater degree. The group tasks could be accomplished, but only at the cost of individual happiness. Freud writes of this in his book *Civilization and Its Discontents* (1930a). Regarding sexuality, he states that for human beings, civilization "… cuts off a fair number of them from sexual enjoyment, and so becomes the source of serious injustice" (p. 104). Freud states that this is necessary, as group members must direct some of their libido toward the group and away from themselves.

With regard to aggression, Freud does not mince words,

> … men are not gentle creatures who want to be loved, and who at the most can defend themselves if they are attacked; they are, on the contrary, creatures among whose instinctual endowments is to be reckoned a powerful share of aggressiveness. As a result, their neighbor is for them not only a potential helper or sexual object, but also someone who tempts them to satisfy their aggressiveness on him, to exploit his capacity for work without compensation, to use him sexually without his consent, to seize his possessions, to humiliate him, to cause him pain, to torture and to kill him. *Homo homini lupus*. Who, in the face of all his experience of life and of history, will have the courage to dispute this assertion? (p. 111)

Being part of a group, however, helps people deal with their aggressive urges. As Freud says,

> It is clearly not easy for men to give up the satisfaction of this inclination to aggression. They do not feel comfortable without it. The advantage which a comparatively small cultural group offers of allowing this instinct an outlet in the form of hostility against intruders is not to be despised. It is always possible to bind together a considerable number of people in love, so long as there are other people left over to receive the manifestations of their aggres-siveness. (p. 114)

As in individual sexual development, group development is governed by a sort of personality organization—not of the individuals but of the group members' relationship with the group leader. In this case, the leader's pathology reflects the group needs.

Knowledge of Freud's group dynamics was expanded by Wilfred Bion, who was a classically trained psychoanalyst. During World War II, Bion was put in charge of developing a selection process for front-line military officers. From this experience, along with his knowledge of psychoanalysis, he conceptualized three types of groups based on *dependency, fight–flight*, and *pairing*. These group types, or "assumptions" as Bion called them, occur in all groups, but become more pronounced in groups that are in crisis or suffering from some sort of breakdown in structure (Bion, 1961).

Dependency group members perceive themselves as weak and inadequate. They are too incompetent and too immature to help the group achieve its goals. Therefore, the group leader is idealized and depended upon to solve the group's problems and attain its goals. The group leader knows all and is infallible. The group members desperately try to extract these qualities of the group leader for themselves and are bound together by their neediness. When the leader fails to live up to the group's unrealistic expectations, they first react with denial and ultimately totally devalue him. The group members then seek out a substitute who can carry the omnipotent projections of the group.

The fight–flight group can be characterized by an *esprit de corps* that relies on the presence of a real or imagined enemy outside of the group. The group shares a common ideology and does not tolerate any deviation. The group is subject to the formation of subgroups that splinter off from the main group. These subgroups cause infighting among the members of the main group. The group as a whole looks to the leader to keep up the fight against perceived outside enemies and to suppress the infighting and splintering into subgroups within the main group. The relationship between the leader and the group members is characterized by control. Either the group is trying to control the leader, or the leader is trying to control the group. There is not much room for middle ground.

The pairing-type group is based upon the projections of the group members onto a couple in the group. The couple symbolizes the ability to procreate and thereby to maintain the integrity of the group. The sexual union of the couple is also seen as something that will save the group from its own internal conflicts, allowing group members to experience intimacy with each other and protection from the hostility and dependency found in the two other types of groups.

We can roughly think of these group types as corresponding to individual personality organization levels. The dependency group is akin to a psychotic personality organization, while the fight–flight type of group, which has many "splitting" aspects among group members and narcissistic qualities among its leaders, resembles borderline and narcissistic personality organizations. Lastly, pairing groups demonstrate the oedipal strivings of the group members and the leaders and resemble a neurotic personality organization.

It should be mentioned that groups can evolve or devolve from one type of group to another or contain the characteristics of more than one group type.

Although Bion's original study was with small groups, his findings have been applied to large groups with success, and his ideas were used by the Tavistock Institute to form intentional training groups, which were the precursor to psychoanalytic therapy groups. The Tavistock groups were characterized by a leader who refused to participate in group decision-making and conflict resolution. Instead, the group leader would (somewhat cryptically) deliver interpretations to the group. The idea was to get the group members to project their anxieties, feelings, and past ways of interacting with authority figures (transference) onto the group leader, who would then, at the appropriate time, "interpret" these processes to the group. This process worked at the Tavistock Institute to elucidate the three different types of groups envisioned by Bion. His ideas about groups are far reaching and still applicable. As organizational development expert Marvin Weisbord (1987) says of Bion's work,

> Keeping people working together instead of fighting or fleeing, seeking to reduce dependency on expert authority and bosses, pushing people to join each other in tasks of mutual importance— these are major consultant contributions to clients buffeted by high-anxiety change. They are, in my opinion, at least as important as the "right answer," since people who are running away, fighting, abdicating, or waiting for a new leader to be born cannot do anything with right answers, even when they have them. (p. 149)

Pressures on group leaders

Otto Kernberg has written about group processes from a psychoanalytic perspective based upon his experience with groups consisting of patients and staff in a hospital setting (Kernberg, 1984b). He identifies several group phenomena such as aggressive and sexual acting out, denial of aggression, depression, and mourning, ascendence of narcissistic and antisocial personalities to leadership positions, as well as intolerance of individual expression. Kernberg has also studied the regressive pressures that act upon group leaders (1980). The isolation of the leader from his peers, the uncertainty about decisions, oedipal fears and frustrations, reduced time for leisure pursuits, and time away from group concerns all create a stressful situation that contributes to the regression of the group leader. According to Kernberg, these regressive pressures can be broken down into the categories of aggression, sexuality, and dependency.

Aggression

Aggressiveness in leaders can be activated by group tensions. The leader is tempted to lash out at the group through the use of authority. This is to be avoided, as it can permanently damage the group structure. The leader must be extremely careful because whatever authority he asserts may be taken out of context and made larger than life by the transference issues within the group. This is especially difficult when the leader has sadistic personality characteristics or the group is of the fight–flight variety. Leaders are always faced with projected aggression because they symbolize a parental image. This is the flip side of the coin to the idealization the leader receives. Like a parent, group leaders engender both parental idealization and rebellious rage from their followers. The projection of aggression onto the group leader by the group serves to emphasize the importance of having a leader with a lack of personal psychopathology. Only an individual with a reasonable personality configuration will have the tolerance for aggression required for good leadership.

Sexuality

The sexuality of the group leader is related to issues of control and power. As mentioned above, the group leader takes on a parental role for the group. Often this is a father figure but can also be a mother figure. The actual gender of the leader may be different from the father or mother figure role they play. The male group leader is unconsciously seen as possessing all the women in the group. Likewise, the reverse holds true when the group leader is a woman. In this case, she is seen as possessing the male group members. These sexual dynamics are a strong source of temptation for the group leader. As Kernberg (1998) says, it is very common to see sexual acting out in the higher levels of a group: "The sexual politics of institutions … are often played out at the top of the institution, as in the proverbial relation between the boss and his secretary or between the chief doctor and head nurse" (p. 63).

In many cases, the unequal sexual relationship between the group leader and a group member serves to play out a sadomasochistic dynamic. The group leader can dominate and control his or her sexual partner, while the sexual partner passively resists by making the group leader feel guilty for his or her domineering behavior. This dynamic is also played out, albeit with a more symbolic sexual aspect, between the group leader and all the group members. The danger in this situation is that the leader's unconscious conflicts can serve to trigger the unconscious conflicts of the group members, leading to a degradation of group functioning and structure.

Another commonly seen aspect of the sexuality of group leaders is a sexual relationship between leaders of the opposite sex. This relationship serves the same function as the pairing group, in which the symbolic pairing of the parental figures of the group serves to defend the group against a regression to a more primitive group organization such as dependency or fight–flight types of groups. However, sexual relations among group leaders carry the danger of a general eroticization of the work environment. This eroticization can inspire increased aggression and a sexualization of group task motivation. In other words, in an eroticized group environment, group members are interested in their roles because of the sexual and aggressive charge they get from being in the group—not because of what they accomplish together as a group. In work groups, this leads to a lack of productivity. This situation can lead to a general breakdown of interpersonal communications in a group. However, when the sexual charge between group members can be controlled and sublimated into the shared work of the group, productive and creative results will accrue. Much of whether the erotic charge in the group is destructive or constructive rests with the maturity of the group leader. This is not to say that successful sexual relationships cannot develop in groups. Nevertheless, when such relationships develop, the structure of the group must accommodate the change. Whether or not the group can do this depends largely on the group leader. Kernberg (1998) describes this as follows: "The main objective of an organization is not to satisfy the human needs of its members, but to carry out a task: one objective of intelligent leadership is to permit the gratification of human needs in carrying out that task" (pp. 66–67).

Dependency

The frustration of dependency needs presents the greatest regressive pressure for the leader. Group members can easily voice their needs to the leader, but the leader cannot reciprocate. Group members can be rewarded for a job well done, while leaders are often overlooked. Of course, group leaders do receive gratification in the sense of the admiration of the group members, successes within their group, and the successful completion of group tasks. Nevertheless, group leaders have few friends or peers to whom they can turn. If a leader turns to a group member, then the group structure and dynamic are distorted, giving rise to many of the same problems caused by sexual relations with group members. It seems that the old proverb is true: It is lonely at the top. The group leader must walk the fine line between being open with group members about his or her needs and letting group members believe that he or she does not require the same gratification as his or her underlings. This also underlines the importance of a consultant to whom the group leader can speak openly and honestly about his or her problems and concerns.

Psychopathology of group leaders

The pressures of aggression, sexuality, and dependency can cause a group leader to regress into a psychopathological state. Although the psychopathology may have been present before the leader took his position, the group leader role greatly increases the pressure toward psychopathology. There are four types of character structures of regressed leaders: *schizoid, obsessive, paranoid,* and *narcissistic.*

The schizoid leader is emotionally isolated and unavailable. This remoteness can frustrate the needs of the group members, causing them to seek out warmth from an intermediate level manager. It is usually these managers who do the actual tasks of leading the group. However, the needs of these managers are also not met, and they are often the first to leave an organization under the control of a schizoid leader.

The obsessive leader is quite common. These leaders are usually orderly, precise, stable, and clear with their instructions. Leaders with these characteristics, however, have their negative side. They may have an excessive need for order and precision, a need not mandated by the group task. Obsessive leaders may also need to maintain strict control over all aspects of the group task, often to the point where they are unable to delegate anything of importance. Such leaders are often unable to tolerate any autonomy or decision-making by group members and will stifle creativity by insisting on a rigid bureaucratic procedure. Because of these characteristics, obsessive leaders often fail to respond to rapidly changing group environments or change that externally impinges on group functioning. This creates unneeded stress during times of transition and change within the group. Obsessive group leaders will also resist change through sadistic acts and attempts to force maintenance of the status quo.

The paranoid leader is suspicious and projects his own rage onto the group. These types of leaders see hidden enemies everywhere and are preoccupied with rooting out the conspiracy in the group. In large-group organizations with multiple levels of hierarchy, such leaders are quick to see many potential hiding places for enemies who are ready to launch an attack. The suppression and eradication of any opposition to these leaders becomes far more important than the group's work task. If paranoid leaders can project their aggression and fears to outside groups, they may be able to function within their own circle. As a result, these types of leaders are most often found in dependency and fight–flight type groups. Nevertheless, since their perceptions of outside groups will be highly distorted, their ability to effectively enable their group to deal constructively with the outside environment is doomed to failure in the long term.

The narcissistic leader is also most often found in dependency and fight–flight type groups. These leaders are grandiose and self-centered. They possess a malignant envy of others, are exceedingly superficial, lack empathy, and have no ability to discern the capabilities of others. Furthermore, when their needs are frustrated, they can easily regress into a paranoid type of leader. Narcissistic leaders are driven by an intense need for power and prestige and are often talented enough, or present themselves as talented enough, to achieve these goals. These leaders foster the dependency needs of the group members in an excessive fashion. In turn, these leaders will devalue group members and ascribe characteristics of inferiority to them. Group members are put into a position in which they must be submissive and passive if they are to receive even the sparsest gratification. Usually, this gratification is doled out as a mirroring of the leader, that is, the leader will praise the group members for being like him or her.

There is a reciprocal relationship between a pathological leader and the organization of group members in that in tightly organized groups the leader may have an outsized effect on the group functioning. As Kernberg (1998) says,

> The more severe the leader's personality pathology and the tighter the organizational structure, the greater are the destructive effects of the leader on the organization. It might be that, under extreme circumstances, the paranoid regression of an entire society maintains the sanity of the tyrant, and, when his control over that society breaks down he becomes psychotic. (p. 96)

There are many examples that support this idea. We could mention Jim Jones and the mass suicide he ordered in Jonestown in 1978, David Koresh and the Branch Davidians' standoff with the FBI in 1993, Joseph Di Mambro and the suicide by fire of the members of the Order of the Solar Temple in Quebec in 1994, and Marshall Applewhite and the mass suicide by Heaven's Gate members in order to reach a spacecraft supposedly hiding in the tail of the Hale-Bopp comet in 1997. Some political upheavals also serve as examples of this leader–group member dynamic. Kernberg (1998) mentions Hitler at the end of the

Nazi regime. We might also suggest the Soviets under Stalin, the North Korean state under the Kims, and perhaps Donald Trump both during and immediately after his presidency in the United States as other examples (K. Volkan, 2021a).

The above conceptualizations of pathological group and leadership processes give an indication of the psychoanalytic understanding of group development. This understanding, however, gives little direct indication of how a psychoanalytic clinician would conduct group psychotherapy. One of the good things about psychotherapy groups is that there is perhaps less chance of the leaders having severe pathologies. The leaders of psychotherapy groups are typically licensed clinicians who have been vetted to some degree by their training and experience. Nevertheless, all group leaders are subject to the influence of group dynamics. The understanding of group structure from a psychoanalytic perspective, therefore, provides a lens for the examination of leadership pathology as well as a critical foundation for making formulations about group process, making formulations about individuals in the groups, and identifying psychotherapeutic interventions that are likely to be effective.

CHAPTER 21

Concepts related to psychoanalytic group psychotherapy

Freud never conducted group psychoanalysis or psychotherapy, and it was left to later clinicians to expand Freud's ideas into group work. For the most part, Freud wrote about naturally forming groups that have emerged in human society. In early human history, these naturally formed groups likely emerged from families and were related to kinship. Over time, group membership began to include others who were geographically close, shared the same language, and shared the same religious and other beliefs. As human communication abilities grew, human groups could become larger. Laws and rules took the place of vigilant leaders or group members on the lookout for "cheaters" (Czárán & Aanen, 2016; Freud, 1912–13). In naturally formed groups, we find the emergence of the types of groups and group leaders discussed above as well as the large-group identifications discussed in a previous chapter. How does all this apply to intentionally formed groups? By intentional groups, we are specifying groups that are brought together for some sort of purpose and would not otherwise naturally emerge. Psychotherapy groups are a good example of this. The construction of an intentional group is artificial. People are brought together by the group leader for a specific reason. That's not to say that the characteristics of natural groups are absent. In fact, all the characteristics of naturally forming groups can be found in intentional groups. The main difference is that the group leader is taking a specific stance in relation to the group. In the history of group psychotherapy, some leaders have fallen sway to their followers' need for omnipotence or have used the group members for their narcissistic or sexual needs. There has been no shortage of psychotherapy, pseudo-psychotherapy, self-help, human potential, and religious counseling groups that demonstrate the pathological qualities of groups mentioned in the last chapter as well as every variety of leadership pathology. Unfortunately, we have seen many such intentional therapeutic groups that are no better than cults. We will leave an exploration of these types of intentional groups for a future piece and focus here on intentional psychoanalytic psychotherapy groups.

Psychoanalytic group psychotherapy

There have been many excellent books written about psychoanalytic or psychodynamic group psychotherapy (e.g., Bateman et al., 2018; Bion, 1961; S. H. Foulkes & Anthony, 1957; E. Foulkes & Pines, 2019; Garland, 2010; König et al., 1994; Kutter, 1982; Pines & Schermer, 1994; Rutan et al., 2014). Since Freud didn't conduct group psychotherapy, psychoanalytically informed group psychotherapy is something that came about without the direct influence of the founder of psychoanalysis. Therefore many different schools and approaches to psychoanalytic or psychodynamic group therapy have been created under the umbrella of psychoanalysis. It is beyond the scope of this book to catalog all these approaches to group psychotherapy or to supply a manual for how to do psychoanalytic group psychotherapy. Many of the authors cited above have explicitly published such guides. Instead, we will describe some important concepts related to group psychotherapy that inform our approach to this therapeutic modality. This approach closely adheres to the psychoanalytic principles we have already outlined. In a way, this "old school" approach to psychoanalytic group psychotherapy will be something new, as most versions of psychoanalytically informed and non-psychoanalytically informed therapy groups emphasize the exploration of relationships. What we will describe is a psychoanalytic group therapy that focuses on patterns of relationships as the outcome of drives and the level of personality organization. This is not much different than how we view individual psychotherapy, with the important exception that the patterns of relationship are more complicated than the dyad between psychotherapist and patient.

Personality organization level and transference in group psychotherapy

As mentioned above, Bion's three group types—dependency, fight–flight, and pairing—can be understood as representing different levels of personality functioning. This is important when considering psychotherapy groups. Bion was one of the first psychoanalysts to form therapy groups. In Bion's groups, the group leader or psychotherapist was strictly neutral, having little interaction with the group members except to give somewhat cryptic interpretations. In modern psychoanalytic group psychotherapy, the psychotherapist group leader maintains analytic neutrality, but interacts with group members more, as in individual psychotherapy, clarifying as well as interpreting resistances, defenses, and transference. Even though there are differences in how group leadership manifests, Bion's ideas or assumptions about groups are applicable to psychoanalytic psychotherapy groups today. Depending on the personality organizational level of the group members, psychotherapy groups will take on the characteristics described by Bion. Psychotherapy groups made up of people functioning with psychotic personality organization will take on the characteristics of dependency groups. Such therapy group members will project a psychoanalytic clinician to be omnipotent, and this group leader will need to provide a holding container for the group members. For this reason, in psychotherapy groups for psychotic individuals, the clinician will typically take on a more supportive and directive role with regard to the group members.

For group members with borderline or narcissistic personality organization, a psychotherapy group will take on the characteristics of fight or flight. Such groups will demonstrate splitting—group members vs. those outside the group, as well as among group members. The psychotherapist in this kind of group must deal with the "us vs. them" mentality of the group as well as mediate aggression between group members. The levels of paranoia and aggression in this kind of a group offer a difficult challenge for the psychotherapist.

Lastly, group members with neurotic personality organization will gravitate toward forming a pairing-type group. This is especially true if the group is run by co-therapists, who will unconsciously take on mother and father roles, though having co-therapists is not necessary. Pairing groups are perhaps the most common type of psychotherapy group, and the group members will deal primarily with oedipal types of conflicts between the group members as well as between the group members and the therapist(s).

S. H. Foulkes (E. Foulkes & Pines, 2019; S. H. Foulkes & Anthony, 1957) posited three types of transference among psychotherapy group members. The first, the central transference, is the transference directed at the psychotherapist group leader. The second type is called a lateral transference, which is transference between members of the group. The third type of transference is transference directed toward the group-as-an-object. Foulkes states that the makeup of a group will determine the nature of the transference in the group. We can extend this idea and state that the type of group, based on Bion's assumptions, can influence each type of transference in psychotherapy groups.

For instance, in groups whose members have psychotic personality organization, the central transference will be emphasized and the lateral transference will be minimized. However, the group-as-an-object transference will be such that identification with the group will provide some support for the reality-testing functions of the group members. It is likely that the central transference of members in such groups will repeatedly expand and contract. The expansion brings a feeling of ambivalent symbiosis with the therapist along with confusion. To defend against the confusion, group members will then pull away from their relationship with the therapist. This expansion and contraction will be repeated until the transference stabilizes (Clarisse et al., 2019).

In fight or flight type groups, where members have borderline or narcissistic personality organization, the central transference will be intense, shifting between positive and negative transference to the psychotherapist group leader. As in individual psychotherapy, the psychotherapy group leader must be able to tolerate the positive and negative transference, projection, and projective identification from group members while maintaining the group as a holding environment. The lateral transference will also oscillate between positive and negative transference among the group members depending on how well the group is doing and whatever is a perceived threat from outside the group. The group-as-an-object transference in the fight or flight type group retains characteristics of splitting as well, with the group being split from perceived enemies or threats from outside the group. When there is a perceived threat from outside the group, members will identify more strongly with the group-as-an-object. In this situation, conflicts between group members will be minimized, and there will be more positive lateral transference. Having an outside "enemy" serves to make the group more cohesive, counteracting threats from outside forces. However, if outside forces overwhelm the group-as-an-object, it can become essentially a "bad" object. Identification with the group-as-an-object will diminish, or group members will take on the "bad" characteristics. In both cases, the lateral transference will become negative. The psychotherapist group leader must try to hold this all together, and, over time, allow for the group members to tolerate aspects within as well as external to the group, allowing the group-as-an-object to become more ambivalent. This is a difficult task for the psychotherapist group leader and may be one of the reasons why in practice we do not see many psychoanalytic therapy groups that are made up of members with borderline or narcissistic personality organization.

In pairing groups, members will typically have neurotic personality organization. Therefore the central transference will be like what is found in individual psychotherapy with people who have this type of personality organization. In pairing groups, the lateral transference is quite strong and often takes on the form of competition for the attention of the psychotherapist group leader(s). There are many vicissitudes to this "sibling" rivalry among pairing group members, including elements of sadomasochism.

"A Child Is Being Beaten" and siblings in the unconscious

Freud's paper "A Child Is Being Beaten" (1919e), based on a series of cases (four women and two men), outlines the development of sadism and masochism among siblings or how pleasure and suffering become linked. Freud reports that around the fifth or sixth year, children start to have fantasies about a child being beaten or punished. This fantasy may be related to seeing a sibling being beaten or disciplined at home. Since children in many cultures typically start going to school around this time, the fantasy is also reinforced by seeing other children being beaten (as used to widely occur) or disciplined by a teacher or other authority figure. The fantasy is related to the Oedipus complex.

The first phase of the fantasy is associated with pleasure and arousal, though this is not yet focused on the genitals. The pleasure comes from watching a rival of whom the child is jealous (typically a sibling) being beaten by the father. This can be actual punishment or the fantasy that the rival is being punished. Initially, the child interprets this as "father loves me and not the child being beaten." This provides sadistic pleasure and is related to the constitution of the individual, not necessarily any traumatic event. Little girls are conscious of the sadistic pleasure in this phase, while boys are not. This sadistic fantasy can be defended against or can last into adulthood, leading to perversion.

In the second phase, both male and female children fantasize about having the exclusive love of the father. In this phase, the child having the fantasy realizes that the child being beaten is getting attention from the father. The child having the fantasy then is jealous of the child being beaten because he or she is getting the love of the father via the beating. In other words, the beating becomes a form of masochistic love. The child feels passively sadistic but then experiences guilt. This leads to repression, causing the child to regress to a sadistic-anal stage where the sadism is transformed into masochism. Due to guilt over the sadistic and incestuous feelings toward the opposite sex parent, the child turns the sadistic feelings toward themselves—that is, masochism, which is also narcissistic. These feelings of sadism and masochism catalyze the third stage. Another perhaps simpler way of thinking of this is that the child feels guilty about the sadistic pleasure he or she derives from seeing the other child being beaten and represses these feelings. However, fantasizing about being loved by the father through getting beaten is not repressed. The experience of masochistic love does not cause repression and feelings of guilt.

In the third phase of the fantasy, the father doing the beating is replaced by a conscious fantasy of another authority figure who is beating someone other than the child (often an anonymous male). In this stage, the child can take both sadistic and masochistic pleasure from the fantasy, identifying with both the beater and the beaten. This fantasy provides sexual excitement that can be gratified through masturbation.

If the oedipal stage is successfully resolved, the "child is being beaten" fantasy loses potency and does not become the primary way adults experience sexual gratification. Sexual deviation usually involves males who presumably have not resolved the oedipal stage of development and who masturbate while having masochistic fantasies. These men transform themselves into part of a woman or they take on a feminine attitude. The person doing the beating becomes a woman—the Oedipus complex is resolved by the boy taking on a feminine role. Then it is the mother who is doing the beating.

The "child is being beaten" fantasy may never completely go away. Although Freud focuses on the sadomasochistic position of the child in the fantasy, another complementary way of viewing the fantasy is by appreciating the gratification experienced through controlling or being in control of another. Modern research has shown that sadomasochistic fantasies and practices are extremely prevalent among human beings. Neuroscientists Ogi Ogas and Sai Gaddam analyzed 500 million sexually relevant Google searches for their book *A Billion Wicked Thoughts* (2011). They found bondage, discipline, sadomasochism (BDSM) subcultures that are widespread and thriving. BDSM fantasies in this subculture can have sexual aspects, but gratification comes mainly from the exercise and exchange of power. Another way of looking at this is that sexual gratification is associated with controlling or being controlled by others. The sadomasochistic impulse is not the only theme of Freud's exposition in "A Child Is Being Beaten," but it indicates more dimensionality to the oedipal situation beyond a child's relationship and identification with parental figures.

We bring this up here because fantasies of controlling and being controlled, this deeper dimension of the oedipal struggle, are commonly experienced in group therapy. Rivalries in groups are not just with the same sex parent but can also be found in those taking on the role of siblings.

As Vamık Volkan and Gabriele Ast have written (1997), there are many different kinds of unconscious fantasies related to a person's siblings during childhood, many of which have the theme of controlling or eliminating the sibling as a rival or an intruder. The most common fantasy concerns the sibling in the mother's belly and consists of controlling the womb so the child can enter it and eliminate the unwanted brother or sister. Another fantasy that is common among younger children is that they are replacements for dead siblings, which we have covered above. Childhood territoriality among siblings can play out in the adult as conditions such as claustrophobia, while other unconscious fantasies related to siblings can manifest in the adult as fear of pregnancy, murderous rage, holiday neuroses, and aberrant identification with siblings. The structure of group psychotherapy allows the rivalries, transferences, and identifications among siblings to be played out in the analytic situation along with the dyadic or triadic transferences with the therapists themselves.

Structure of a psychoanalytic therapy group

Regarding the structure and conduct of a psychoanalytic psychotherapy group, we have found that the guidance that has worked best for us adheres fairly closely to what was described by the psychoanalyst S. H. Foulkes. His psychoanalytic approach to group psychotherapy evolved from his experience creating therapy groups during World War II. Foulkes (E. Foulkes & Pines, 2019) describes what he calls group analysis like this:

> Group analysis, as I understand it, works on the group model. Many of its processes we know from the two-personal situation, but with the additional features that can be seen in full in interaction between two, three or more persons. They can be seen as what they are—interactional processes, not processes in the isolated individual. In addition to this we can make observations that are concealed in the one- or two-personal situation and thus discover group-specific factors in operation. (p. 156)

Here, Foulkes indicates the further dimensionality provided by the interactions of more than two individuals in a group. He sees the emergence of the perspective of the group-as-an-object as the central advantage of group psychotherapy.

Foulkes proposes several general guidelines for psychoanalytic group psychotherapy. To begin with, he recommends that patients for group therapy be derived by referrals from the practices of different psycho-analysts or psychotherapists. In our experience, these external referrals are usually augmented by referring one's own individual psychoanalytic or psychotherapy patients to the group. Having one's own individual patients in a group can be a disadvantage because the clinician knows these patients better than those referred by someone else. Group psychotherapy patients will pick up the fact that the therapist already has a closer relationship with his or her individual patients, and this can generate jealousy. However, any perceived favoritism is just grist for the mill to be worked through as part of the group process. From the point of view of maintaining a modern psychotherapy practice, psychoanalytic clinicians perhaps cannot be as choosy as Foulkes about where their group therapy patients come from. Also, patients coming to a group often will bring in "built-in" transferences that must be worked through, which can slow the development of group cohesiveness.

Foulkes also recommends that patients be somewhat homogeneous regarding demographic and socioeconomic factors as well as level of intelligence and insight. In general, homogeneity in these factors makes leading the psychotherapy group easier for the clinician. Insight is related to the patient's level of personality organization, and as explained in more detail below, homogeneity is desirable to increase group functioning. Foulkes does not consider this to be important, but this is likely because the members of his group were functioning at a similar level of personality organization. What we can say is that specific diagnoses, within a level of personality functioning, are not an important consideration in group membership.

The history of psychotherapy indicates that it has been biased toward the values of the majority culture—in the United States, this would be white middle-class culture. It is no surprise that many people from nonwhite ethnic groups are distrustful or dismissive of psychotherapy. Because of this, we advocate for some heterogeneity in group members' demographic characteristics. This requires both the clinician and group members to learn about cultures and values different than their own. We have seen this have a powerful effect in group therapy settings, and it is well worth the extra effort on behalf of the clinician.

Psychoanalytic psychotherapy groups can be open or closed. Membership in closed groups is set in the beginning and remains the same, with no new members being added. These groups usually run for a predetermined amount of time—for example, six months, two years, etc. In modern times, this type of group is not often seen in treatment groups but is commonly seen in psychotherapy training groups. Closed groups are not realistic regarding maintaining a practice where having the ability to add members and keep a group running has important clinical and financial consequences. Open-ended groups, or what Foulkes called slow-open groups, are groups that run for an indeterminate amount of time—sometimes for years—with members transiting in and out. This kind of group is the most common type of psychodynamic psychotherapy group. With open-ended groups, an important question is how to bring in new members, especially if the group has been running for a while. In practice, psychoanalytic psychotherapy groups are often semi-open, meaning that the membership is kept fairly stable for a period of time, say a year, without bringing in new members. In this type of group, new members are brought in only after a current member has terminated therapy and left the group. The timing and introduction of new group members must be facilitated with care. In our experience, this seems to provide the stability and consistency of closed groups while allowing the flexibility of open groups.

We consider that the psychoanalytic therapy group should have between five and eight patients. Foulkes recommends eight patients as the ideal, with equal numbers of men and women. In our experience, groups with men and women in roughly equal numbers work well. However, same gender groups of all women or all men also work well and may work better for groups made up of people whose personality organization has not reached the neurotic level. Another way of thinking of this is that you can mix genders, or you can mix personality organization level, but not both. Transgender people may be part of mixed groups. Transgender and nonbinary individuals may also join a same gender group that is closest to their gender identification or separate groups can be set up for transgender or nonbinary individuals. The same can be said for LGBTQ+ people, though general psychoanalytic group therapy does not specifically focus on LGBTQ+ issues. Nevertheless, in groups comprised of LGBTQ+ individuals, these issues will no doubt arise.

Groups can be started with fewer, say three to four, patients, but more patients should be added to the group as soon as possible before it group becomes cohesive. Having more than eight patients in a group becomes problematic for the psychotherapist, who must keep track of the complicated dynamics related to her- or himself and the group members, and the patterns of relationship among the group members. In our experience, even having eight group members is a bit unwieldy, with six to seven patients being ideal.

Psychoanalytic group members should ideally not know one another well or have any sort of preexisting relationship. This helps tremendously to keep the transference relationships in the group clear and to avoid any acting out. This can be considered as therapeutic abstinence. Foulkes also avoids interacting with patients outside group sessions to maintain a psychoanalytic stance toward group patients. This includes not doing individual psychoanalysis or psychotherapy with group members. This is probably best in an ideal situation but is rarely practical. In our experience, some patients continue to receive individual psychotherapy as well as group psychotherapy simultaneously. This is especially important for patients who are not functioning at a neurotic level of personality organization and who may therefore need more therapeutic containment. There is also the consideration that clinicians in private practice do not want to give up the income derived from seeing patients in individual psychotherapy. As mentioned, it is likely that patients seeing their clinician in individual sessions will engender jealousy and rivalry among other group members who are only in group psychotherapy. The jealousies and rivalries are very important to work with because they represent transferences that need to be resolved. In practice, we have found this sort of jealousy over what is perceived as extra attention from the clinician (as a parental figure) to be quite common. If such jealousy and rivalry, as well as fantasies related to this, are not brought to light during the group sessions, it can engender acting out outside of the group.

In general, it is best if the level of personality organization among the group members is roughly the same. Neurotic level personality organization patients will get the most from being in a psychotherapy group. Group psychotherapy is fertile ground for experiencing the full spectrum of oedipal conflicts, but the patients should be ready to engage with these. Patients with more primitive personality organization that are mixed in with patients functioning at a neurotic level of personality organization will attempt to "reach up" and engage in oedipal struggles. However, their oedipal strivings will be tinged with amounts of aggression toward other group members, and such patients will focus on the relationship (the dyad) between themselves and the therapist. Just as in individual psychotherapy, this dyadic relationship between the therapist and group member with more primitive personality organization will take on the characteristics of the personality level of the patient—splitting defenses, narcissistic responses, or disorganization. The group member with a more primitive personality organization will often become frustrated that they are not receiving most of the attention from the therapist. This will unconsciously lead him or her to act out in ways that will gain them more attention. This can be extremely disruptive to the group process. Neurotic level personality organization group members will become overwhelmed by the acting out of the more primitive level group member and will shut down psychologically, as one of Kevin Volkan's cases exemplifies.

Case example of acting out

Sally, a thirty-six-year-old woman with a diagnosis of bipolar disorder, was invited to join an ongoing psychoanalytic psychotherapy group by her psychotherapist, who co-led the therapy group with me. Sally, who was well educated and articulate at first, seemed uneasy upon joining the group. She rarely interacted with other members of the group, and when she did, she was often hostile. Over time, it was apparent that Sally had other issues besides her bipolar diagnosis. She reported that her relationships were unstable and that she had problems with alcohol and psychoactive prescription drugs such as Xanax.

In the group sessions, Sally would only speak to me and ignore the female co-therapist. She appeared to crave my attention for much of the session. If group members tried to speak to me, Sally would become hostile toward them. After a while, the group members became reticent to confront Sally. When I brought this to Sally's attention, she vigorously denied monopolizing my time. At the next session, Sally was openly hostile toward me and would only speak to my co-therapist. The following week, this dynamic reversed itself. Over several sessions, Sally would flip back and forth between talking to me or my co-therapist. While other group members would assert themselves to work with me or the co-therapist, these conversations had a dyadic feel to them, and there was little interaction between the group members.

After a few months of this, Sally overdosed on Xanax and had to be hospitalized. We held group therapy sessions without her, during which there was much more interaction among group members. Transference manifestations among group members suddenly seemed to appear, whereas before, the transference seemed to exist solely between myself and the co-therapist. After being released from the hospital, Sally decided not to return to the therapy group but continued working with my colleague in individual therapy. Without Sally present, the group functioning appeared to improve almost immediately. Sibling rivalries that group members had been too timid to express suddenly started making appearances.

This case fragment illustrates some of the pitfalls of mixing people with differing personality organization into the same group.

As mentioned above, our view is that psychoanalytic group therapy should ideally be conducted by male and female co-therapists. This allows for the full expression of transference to both mother and father figures in the group. However, this is not a hard and fast requirement, and a lone therapist of any gender may successfully run a psychoanalytic therapy group. Two therapists of the same gender can also successfully facilitate psychoanalytic therapy groups. If there are co-therapists, it is important for them to share insights and formulations about group members. A consistent approach to each group member by both therapists vastly strengthens the effectiveness of the therapy. In our experience, coming to agree on a formulation for each group member, and the sharing of countertransference reactions and counterresponses between the co-therapists, helps to blunt the effect of projective identification on to either or both therapists, as well as helping the therapists to make more insightful interpretations.

Foulkes recommends that psychoanalytic psychotherapy groups meet twice a week for an hour and a half. In our experience, this allows for intensive therapeutic work to take place relatively quickly. However, once a week groups meeting for an hour and a half work just fine, though the intensity of the group process may take longer to build up. Group psychotherapy needs more than the regular fifty-minute therapeutic hour, and the rhythm of group sessions is different than individual psychoanalysis or psychotherapy sessions. Kevin Volkan has experience with several group psychotherapy configurations ranging from those that ran from an hour a week to marathon group sessions that went sixteen hours over a weekend. In his opinion, an hour and a half seems about right, though two-hour sessions can also work well for weekly groups. It would be interesting to experiment with doing marathon psychoanalytic groups; however, the problem with longer group configurations is that it becomes difficult for the therapist to maintain strict neutrality over such a long period of time.

With regard to the psychoanalytic group psychotherapy setting, it is fairly typical of group therapy in general. There are seats arranged in a circle so that all members face each other and the therapist(s). When there are two co-therapists, we have found that having them sit next to each other or on opposite sides of the room is best. This can be varied across sessions; however, where the co-therapists sit will feed into the group members' transference and fantasies about the therapists. For instance, if the therapists are sitting apart, group members may fantasize that the co-therapists (mom and dad) are fighting. Typically, where group members sit during any given session is not assigned beforehand. Group therapists can gain a good deal of insight into how the group as a whole and individual members are doing by noticing where people sit. When a therapy group is first formed, members will sit in different places. After a while, members will gravitate toward sitting in the same place for each session and a seating pattern will emerge. When the seating pattern is disrupted—such as when someone sits in a different seat—this can be seen as a form of acting out. This acting out could be due to a rivalry or transference manifestation and should be noted by the therapist(s) but not necessarily immediately commented on to the group. This is a good opportunity for the therapist(s) to observe changes in group dynamics. Allowing the situation to mature on its own may give even more insight into the unconscious processes among the group members.

Overall, group psychotherapy should have

> ... a minimum of directions and guidance regarding behavior and content ... The analytical approach is above all introduced by the conductor, by his own analytical attitude, which in all essentials is analogous to that of the psychoanalyst in the psychoanalytical situation. The analyst in the group can be more natural and personal than in the psychoanalytical situation. It needs particular qualifications and experience to remain at the same time sufficiently detached so as not to impede transference needs. He allows the group members free expression of their personal involvement and interpretations of his actions, and accepts them as expressions of transference. Everything under observation is taken as communication, whether verbal or nonverbal behavior, and therefore in need of interpretation. This rests on the notion that everything can be taken as an associative response, a reaction against or an unconscious interpretation of what was happening. Everything is seen as meaningful in the light of the total context of the group. (E. Foulkes & Pines, 2019, p. 172)

Psychoanalytic psychotherapy groups need little structure, and the group psychotherapist (labeled as a conductor by Foulkes) should approach group psychoanalytic therapy like individual psychoanalytic psychotherapy. The psychotherapist should actively interpret defenses and resistances, and later, transferences—especially compulsively repeated transferences that derive from early childhood. However, without compromising neutrality, the therapist may function with a bit more openness. Foulkes (E. Foulkes & Pines, 2019) has observed that group members often connect unconscious content related to what is going on in the group sessions to their own current life situations, as well as impactful childhood experiences. Group therapy will not work in as great detail with infantile transference neuroses as psychoanalysis or even psychoanalytic psychotherapy. However, attention to where members' current life events connect to what goes on in the group sessions can yield valuable information about unconscious conflicts in the group. "Timely attention to this area prevents much unnecessary acting out, or living through, and helps to concentrate all relevant meaning in the treatment situation" (p. 173).

While psychoanalytic therapy groups can continue indefinitely, individual group members typically stay with a group for between two and four years. Members of twice weekly groups may unsurprisingly make quicker progress than members of once-a-week groups, but this is not always the case, and therapeutic progress is dependent on many other factors as well. We have noticed that when patients become ripe for termination from group therapy the group almost runs itself, with the therapist(s) needing little intervention. Patients begin to make interpretations to each other and themselves and respond to these insights in a mature and thoughtful manner. It becomes clear when a patient has internalized awareness of his or her transference patterns, resistances, and defenses, when they insightfully comment on these before the therapist has a chance to say anything! As in individual psychoanalytic psychotherapy, termination can be planned and issues around it worked on. We have found that two to four months seem to be on average enough time for proper termination from a psychoanalytic psychotherapy group. Unlike individual psychotherapy, termination from group psychotherapy must consider the ending of more relationships than that of the therapist(s)–patient dyad or triad. Changes in relationships among group members as well as changes in the group identity must be processed. These changes will need to be considered even after a patient leaves the group and will affect the introduction of new members into the group as well. There seems to be a rhythm to when it is time for a patient to terminate, as if there are certain optimal inflection points. As Foulkes says,

> A "spiral notion" seems to apply—that is, that at various times we arrive at a favorable moment for concluding treatment; if these points are missed, we have to count on a longer period until such a point is reached again. The experienced group analyst can assess fairly accurately when such an extension is worthwhile. (p. 174)

Psychoanalytic group psychotherapy can induce permanent insight into one's own unconscious conflicts as well as help facilitate positive relationships with others, especially with intimate partners and authority figures. Psychoanalytic group psychotherapy is also very practical. Over the years, psychoanalysis has been criticized for the elite nature of its patients—people who can afford multiple sessions each week over many years. Psychoanalytic psychotherapy to a lesser degree is similarly available to those with time and money. Group psychoanalytic psychotherapy does not have this problem. It is inexpensive and available to people with modest incomes. It is also as effective as any other type of psychotherapy and capable of bringing about positive change in the lives of people who might not otherwise be able to experience the benefits of psychotherapy.

Coda

Although there are textbooks on psychoanalysis and psychoanalytic psychotherapy, developments in psychoanalytic findings and theories warranted a new volume that would include these findings while maintaining the necessary principles that have stood the test of time. In this book, we have looked at several new developments in particular.

- *First*, many patients with low-level personality organization now seek psychoanalytic treatment. Therefore we have included information about, and examples of, different personality organizations throughout this book. It is imperative to evaluate our patients' internal psychological structures at the beginning of therapeutic work to modify classical technical steps while we are treating individuals with low-level personality organization.
- *Second*, while everyone has unconscious fantasies, in this book we have described how some events in childhood may "actualize" such fantasies. We describe how dealing with unconscious fantasies that are actualized requires special attention.
- The *third* one is our deeper understanding of the influence shared external events have in shaping symptom and personality formation. While working with our patients we are now more

aware of the intertwining of external and internal events and large-group identity and cultural issues.

- *Fourth* is the exploration of transgenerational transmission of trauma that has taught psychoanalytic clinicians how historical traumatic events that took place in the lives of a person's ancestors sometimes play a role in structuring this individual's internal world.

- *Fifth*, the concept of "action" in psychoanalysis has been expanded from being simply considered unwanted "acting out." We now appreciate that a certain type of patients' activities that we have named "therapeutic play" is part of the healing process.

- *Sixth*, psychoanalytic clinicians now pay more attention to their counterresponses and countertransference to their patients, and search for ways to utilize such responses therapeutically.

- *Seventh*, our profession has seen a growing "pluralism" and many new schools in psychoanalysis. This development questions some old considerations and suggests new ones. Nevertheless, generally speaking, it also creates confusion about theory and technique. We kept this in mind while writing this book and have tried to reduce any confusion in the reader's mind by not focusing on any one psychoanalytic school. Drawing upon our years of experience, experiences of biculturalism, and our experiences supervising younger psychoanalytic clinicians in various countries and cultures, we have presented case examples illustrating technical issues that refer to the contemporary ideas listed above, while holding on to classical and still necessary technical tools.

- *Eighth*, an understanding of group processes has allowed us a way to see how psychoanalytic principles play out in social and organizational settings. Insight from a psychoanalytic understanding of groups has allowed for the development of psychoanalytic group psychotherapy, the principles of which we have outlined here. This type of psychoanalytic therapy is accessible to almost anyone who wants or needs to do therapeutic work, while at the same time proving extremely effective.

All the points above should remind us that psychoanalysis and psychoanalytic psychotherapy are living professions. Keeping this in mind counteracts the tendency to enshrine and dogmatize past theory and technique into a sort of manualized form of therapy. Instead, we can build upon valid psychoanalytic knowledge and expand the reach of our theory and practice into new areas while improving our ability to help others.

Psychoanalysis and psychoanalytic psychotherapy require that the practitioner has the ability to improvise and deal with the unexpected. As Howard Bacal and Bruce Herzog (2003) write,

> Regardless of whether an analytic event was intentional, any interaction can still have therapeutic potential. This supposition allows for the efficacy of surprise, spontaneity, and improvisation in the analytic encounter. Therefore, all spontaneously occurring interactions should be given serious consideration by the therapist as to their mutative potential. (p. 644)

Going into the future, it is imperative that we do not lose this aspect of psychoanalytic clinical work. We live in an era when new technical approaches such as "shuttle analysis," including telephone, Skype, and Zoom, as well as similar online modalities, are being used to meet with patients online instead of in a traditional office setting. Many of us have also been supervising our students and trainees using these online modalities. These changes have been driven by the Covid-19 pandemic and the advent of new technology. Our concern is that the use of online modalities will diminish the kind of human contact necessary for spontaneous, improvisatory psychoanalytic practices, rendering our therapeutic work less effective. We continue to adhere to the belief that after the viral pandemic is over, the best way to conduct psychoanalysis and psychoanalytic psychotherapy is to see patients in our offices. Nevertheless, we understand that many psychoanalytic clinicians may prefer to remain online with their work. This is because of ease of patient access, reduced practice associated costs, and the ability to expand one's practice beyond geographic limitations—all legitimate reasons. Since online practice is relatively new, it is our hope that innovations in technology and therapeutic technique will be able to maintain the vital living nature of psychoanalytic work along with the human contact that is so significant to our patients. It is important to remember the need to protect the basic principles of psychoanalytic-based treatment carefully even as the manner in which we deliver treatment changes.

References

Abend, S. M. (1990). Unconscious fantasies and theories of cure. *Journal of the American Psychoanalytic Association, 27*: 579–596.

Abend, S. M. (2008). Unconscious fantasy and modern conflict theory. *Psychoanalytic Inquiry, 28*: 117–130.

Abraham, K. (1924). The influence of oral eroticism in character formation. In: *Selected Papers of Karl Abraham. M. D.* (pp. 393–406). New York: Brunner/Mazel.

Adler, E., & Bachant, L. (1996). Free association and analytic neutrality: The basic structure of the psychoanalytic situation. *American Journal of Psychoanalysis, 44*: 1021–1046.

Agatsuma, S. (2014). Differentiating two kinds of neutrality. *International Forum of Psychoanalysis, 23*: 238–245.

Ainslie, R. C., & Solyom, A. E. (1986). The replacement of the fantasied oedipal child: A disruptive effect of sibling loss on the mother–infant relationship. *Psychoanalytic Psychology, 3*: 257–268.

Akhtar, S. (2000). From schisms through synthesis to informed oscillation: An attempt at integrating some diverse aspects of psychoanalytic technique. *Psychoanalytic Quarterly, 69*: 265–288.

Akhtar, S. (2009). *Comprehensive Dictionary of Psychoanalysis*. London: Karnac.

Alexander, F., & French, T. M. (1946). *Psychoanalytic Therapy: Principles and Application*. New York: Ronald.

Anzieu, D. (1984). *The Group and the Unconscious.* London: Routledge & Kegan Paul.

Arlow, J. A. (1969). Unconscious fantasy and disturbances of conscious experience. *Psychoanalytic Quarterly, 38*: 1–27.

Arlow, J. A. (1979). Genesis of interpretation. *Journal of the American Psychoanalytic Association, 27* (suppl.): 193–206.

Bacal, H., & Herzog, B. (2003). Specificity theory and optimal responsiveness: An outline. *Psychoanalytic Psychology, 20*: 635–648.

Bateman, A., Brown, D., & Pedder, J. (2018). *Introduction to Psychotherapy: An Outline of Psychodynamic Principles and Practice.* London: Routledge.

Beres, D. (1962).The unconscious fantasy. *Psychoanalytic Quarterly, 31*: 309–329.

Berger, E. U. (2016). *Toward an Integration of Cognitive Behavioral Therapy and Psychodynamic Treatment for Survivors of Sexual Trauma: A Critical Review of the Literature.* Ann Arbor, MI: ProQuest Information & Learning.

Bergmann, M. V. (1982). Thoughts on super-ego pathology of survivors and their children. In: M. S. Bergmann & M. E. Jucovy (Eds.), *Generations of the Holocaust* (pp. 287–311). New York: Basic Books.

Berne, E. (1961). *Transactional Analysis in Psychotherapy: A Systematic Individual and Social Psychiatry.* New York: Grove.

Bibring, E. (1954). Psychoanalysis and dynamic psychotherapies. *Journal of the American Psychoanalytic Association, 2*: 745–746.

Bion, W. R. (1961). *Experiences in Groups.* New York: Basic Books.

Blackman, J. S. (2004). *101 Defenses: How the Mind Shields Itself.* New York: Routledge.

Blackman, J. S. (2020). A psychoanalytic view of reactions to the coronavirus pandemic in China. *American Journal of Psychoanalysis, 80*: 119–132.

Blackman, J. S., & Dring, K. (2022). *Developmental Evaluation of Children and Adolescents: A Psychodynamic Guide.* New York: Routledge.

Blass, R. (2003). On ethical issues at the foundation of the debate over the goals of psychoanalysis. *International Journal of Psychoanalysis, 84*: 929–944.

Bloom, P. (2010). *How Pleasure Works: The New Science of Why We Like What We Like.* New York: W. W. Norton.

Blos, P. (1966). *On Adolescence: A Psychoanalytic Interpretation.* New York: Free Press.

Blos, P. (1979). *The Adolescence Passage: Developmental Issues.* New York: International Universities Press.

Blum, H. P. (1985). Superego formation, adolescent transformation and the adult neurosis. *Journal of the American Psychoanalytic Association, 4*: 887–909.

Blum, H. P. (2003). Psychoanalytic controversies: Repression, transference and reconstruction. *International Journal of Psychoanalysis, 84*: 497–513.

Böhm, T. (2002). Reflections on psychoanalytic listening. *Scandinavian Psychoanalytic Review, 25*: 20–26.

Bornstein, M. (1983). Values and neutrality in psychoanalysis. *Psychoanalytic Inquiry, 3*: 547–717.

Boss, J. M. (1979). The seventeenth-century transformation of the hysteric affection, and Sydenham's Baconian medicine. *Psychological Medicine, 9*: 221–234.

Bowlby, J. (1958). The nature of the child's tie to his mother. *International Journal of Psychoanalysis, 39*: 350–373.

Bowlby, J. (1960). Separation anxiety. *International Journal of Psychoanalysis, 41*: 89–113.

Bowlby, J. (1978). Attachment theory and its therapeutic implications. *Adolescent Psychiatry, 6*: 5–33.

Boyer, L. B. (1983). *The Regressed Patient.* New York: Jason Aronson.

Boyer, L. B. (1999). *Countertransference and Regression.* Northvale, NJ: Jason Aronson.

Brenner, C. (1979). Working alliance, therapeutic alliance and transference. *Journal of the American Psychoanalytic Association, 27*: 137–157.

Brenner, I. (2001). *Dissociation of Trauma: Theory, Phenomenology, and Technique.* Madison, CT: International Universities Press.

Brenner, I. (2004). *Psychic Trauma: Dynamics, Symptoms, and Treatment.* New York: Jason Aronson.

Brenner, I. (Ed.) (2019). *The Handbook of Psychoanalytic Holocaust Studies: International Perspectives.* New York: Routledge.

Bromberg, N. (1971). Hitler: Hitler's character and its development: Further observations. *American Imago, 28*: 289–303.

Brown, C., & Lewis, M. J. (2003). Psychosocial development in the elderly: An investigation into Erikson's ninth state. *Journal of Aging Studies, 17*: 415–426.

Budak, M. U. (2015). The replacement child syndrome following stillbirth: A reconsideration. *Enfance Psychologie, Pédagogie, Neuropsychiatrie, Sociologie, 3*: 351–364.

Cain, A. C., & Cain, B. S. (1964). On replacing a child. *Journal of the American Academy of Child Psychiatry, 3*: 443–456.

Cameron, N. (1961). Introjection, reprojection, and hallucination in the interaction between schizophrenic patient and therapist. *International Journal of Psychoanalysis, 42*: 86–96.

Carroll, S. (2022). Frans de Waal on culture and gender in primates (No. 194). Retrieved April 25 from https://preposterousuniverse.com/podcast/2022/04/25/194-frans-de-waal-on-culture-and-gender-in-primates/

Chasseguet-Smirgel, J. (1984). *The Ego Ideal.* New York: W. W. Norton.

Chodorow, N. (1978a). *The Reproduction of Mothering: Psychoanalysis and the Sociology of Gender.* Berkeley, CA: University of California Press.

Chodorow, N. (1978b). Mothering, object-relations, and the female oedipal configuration. *Feminist Studies, 4*: 137–158.

Clarisse, V., Guy, G., & Bonnet, C. (2019). The psychotic transference in groups. *Group Analysis, 52*: 491–502.

Cooper, A. M. (1989). Narcissism and masochism: The narcissistic-masochistic character. *Psychiatric Clinics of North America, 12*: 541–552.

Czárán, T., & Aanen, D. K. (2016). The early evolution of cooperation in humans: On cheating, group identity and group size. *Behaviour, 153*: 1247–1266.

De Angel, L., & Turek, L. (1990). Observaciones sobre la transferencia en el hospital de día (Observations on transformations in a day hospital). *Clínica y Análisis Grupal, 12*: 273–281.

Dewald, P. A., & Clark, R. W. (Eds.) (2001). *Ethics Case Book of the American Psychoanalytic Association.* New York: American Psychoanalytic Association.

DiGiorgio, K. E., Arnkoff, D. B., Glass, C. R., Lyhus, K. E., & Walter, R. C. (2004). EMDR and theoretical orientation: A qualitative study of how therapists integrate eye movement desensitization and reprocessing into their approach to psychotherapy. *Journal of Psychotherapy Integration, 14*: 227–252.

Dunbar, R. I. M. (1993). Coevolution of neocortical size, group size and language in humans. *Behavioral and Brain Sciences, 16*: 681–735. https://doi.org/10.1017/S0140525X00032325

Emde, R. N. (1988a). Development terminable and interminable, I: Innate and motivational factors from infancy. *International Journal of Psychoanalysis, 69*: 23–42.

Emde, R. N. (1988b). Development terminable and interminable, II: Recent psychoanalytic theory and therapeutic considerations. *International Journal of Psychoanalysis, 69*: 283–296.

Emde, R. N. (1991). Positive emotions for psychoanalytic theory: Surprises from infancy research and new directions. *Journal of the American Psychoanalytic Association* (Supplement), *39*: 5–44.

Erikson, E. H. (1950). *Childhood and Society.* New York: W. W. Norton.

Erikson, E. H. (1956). The problem of ego identity. *Journal of the American Psychoanalytic Association, 4*: 56–121.

Erikson, E. H. (1959). *Identity and the Life Cycle*. New York: International Universities Press.

Erikson, E. H. (1968). *Identity, Youth and Crisis*. New York: W. W. Norton.

Faimberg, H. (2005). *The Telescoping of Generations: Listening to the Narcissistic Links Between Generations*. London: Routledge.

Fairbairn, W. R. D. (1958). On the nature and aims of psycho-analytical treatment. *International Journal of Psychoanalysis, 39*: 374–385.

Ferenczi, S. (2012). *Final Contributions to the Problems and Methods of Psycho-Analysis*. London: Karnac.

Fonagy, P. (1999). Memory and therapeutic action. *International Journal of Psychoanalysis, 80*: 215–223.

Fonagy, P., & Target, M. (1997). Attachment and reflective functions: Their role in self-organization. *Developmental Psychopathology, 9*: 679–700.

Fonagy, P., & Target, M. (1998). Mentalization and the changing aim of child analysis. *Psychoanalytic Dialogues, 8*: 87–114.

Foulkes, E., & Pines, M. (Eds.) (2019). *Selected Papers of S. H. Foulkes: Psychoanalysis and Group Analysis*. New York: Routledge.

Foulkes, S. H., & Anthony, E. J. (1957). *Group Psychotherapy: The Psycho-Analytic Approach*. New York: Penguin.

Fox, A. (2018). Gay-friendly psychoanalysis and the abiding pleasures of prejudice. *Studies in Gender and Sexuality, 19*: 265–278.

Freud, A. (1936). *The Ego and the Mechanisms of Defense*. New York: International Universities Press.

Freud, A. (1954). The widening scope of indications for psychoanalysis. In: *The Writings of Anna Freud, Vol. 4* (pp. 356–376). New York: International Universities Press, 1968.

Freud, A. (1968). *The Writings of Anna Freud. Vol. 1–4*. New York: International Universities Press.

Freud, A., & Burlingham, D. (1942). *War and Children*. New York: International Universities Press.

Freud, A., Nagera, H., & Freud, W. E. (1965). Metapsychological assessment of the adult's personality: The adult profile. *Psychoanalytic Study of the Child, 20*: 9–14.

Freud, S. (1895d). *Studies On Hysteria* (with J. Breuer). *S. E.*, 2: 19–312. London: Hogarth.

Freud, S. (1900a). *The Interpretation of Dreams. S. E.*, 4–5: ix–627. London: Hogarth.

Freud, S, (1905d). *Three Essays on the Theory of Sexuality. S. E.*, 7: 130–242. London: Hogarth.

Freud, S. (1908a). Hysterical phantasies and their relation to bisexuality. *S. E.*, 9: 155–166. London: Hogarth.

Freud, S. (1909b). Analysis of a phobia in a five-year-old boy. *S. E.*, *10*: 3–148. London: Hogarth.

Freud, S. (1909c). Family romances. *S. E.*, *9*: 237–241. London: Hogarth.

Freud, S. (1909d). Notes upon a case of obsessional neurosis. *S. E.*, *10*: 155–320. London: Hogarth.

Freud, S. (1911c). Psychoanalytic notes on an autobiographical account of a case of paranoia (Dementia paranoides). *S. E.*, *12*: 9–80. London: Hogarth.

Freud, S. (1912e). Recommendations to physicians practising psycho-analysis. *S. E.*, *12*: 109–120. London: Hogarth.

Freud, S. (1912–13). *Totem and Taboo*. Resemblances between the psychic lives of savages and neurotics. *S. E.*, *13*: vii–162. London: Hogarth.

Freud, S. (1914c). On narcissism. *S. E.*, *14*: 67–103. London: Hogarth.

Freud, S. (1914d). On the history of the psycho-analytic movement. *S. E.*, *14*: 1–66. London: Hogarth.

Freud, S. (1914g). Remembering, repeating and working-through). *S. E.*, *12*: 145–156. London: Hogarth.

Freud, S. (1915a). Observations on transference-love (further recommendations on the technique of psycho-analysis, III). *S. E.*, *12*: 157–171. London: Hogarth.

Freud, S. (1918b). *From the History of an Infantile Neurosis*. *S. E.*, *17*: 1–124. London: Hogarth.

Freud, S. (1919a). Lines of advance in psycho-analytic therapy. *S. E.*, *17*: 157–168. London: Hogarth.

Freud, S. (1919e). "A child is being beaten". A contribution to the study of the origin of sexual perversions. *S. E.*, *17*: 175–204. London: Hogarth.

Freud, S. (1920g). *Beyond the Pleasure Principle*. *S. E.*, *18*: 3–64. London: Hogarth.

Freud, S. (1921c). *Group Psychology and the Analysis of the Ego*. *S. E.*, *18*: 65–144. London: Hogarth.

Freud, S. (1923b). *The Ego and the Id*. *S. E.*, *19*: 1–66. London: Hogarth.

Freud, S. (1923e). The infantile genital organization. *S. E.*, *19*: 141–145. London: Hogarth.

Freud, S. (1924c). The economic problem of masochism. *S. E.*, *19*: 157–170. London: Hogarth.

Freud, S. (1925j). Some psychical consequences of the anatomical distinction between the sexes. *S. E.*, *19*: 241–258. London: Hogarth.

Freud, S. (1926e). *The Question of Lay Analysis*. *S. E.*, *20*: 177–258. London: Hogarth.

Freud, S. (1926d). *Inhibitions, Symptoms and Anxiety. S. E., 20*: 75–175. London: Hogarth.

Freud, S. (1930a). *Civilization and Its Discontents. S. E., 21*: 57–146. London: Hogarth.

Freud, S. (1933a). *New Introductory Lectures on Psycho-Analysis. S. E., 22*: 7–182. London: Hogarth.

Freud, S. (1937c). Analysis terminable and interminable. *S. E., 23*: 209–253. London: Hogarth.

Freud, S. (1940a [1938]). An outline of psycho-analysis. *S. E., 23*: 139–208. London: Hogarth.

Freud, S. (1941e). Address to the Society of *B'nai B'rith. S. E., 20*: 271–274. London: Hogarth.

Fromm-Reichmann, F. (1950). *Principles of Intensive Psychotherapy*. Chicago, IL: University of Chicago Press.

Gabbard, G. O. (2004). *Long-Term Psychodynamic Psychotherapy: A Basic Text*. Washington, DC: American Psychiatric Publishing.

Garland, C. (2010). Psychoanalytic group therapy with severely disturbed patients: Benefits and challenges. In: P. Williams (Ed.), *The Psychoanalytic Therapy of Severe Disturbance* (pp. 81–102). London: Karnac.

Garrett, M. (2019). *Psychotherapy for Psychosis: Integrating Cognitive-Behavioral and Psychodynamic Treatment*. New York: Guilford.

Gelso, C. J., & Kanninen, K. M. (2017). Neutrality revisited: On the value of being neutral within an empathic atmosphere. *Journal of Psychotherapy Integration, 27*: 330–341.

Gill, M. (1994). *Psychoanalysis in Transition: A Personal View*. Hillsdale, NJ: Analytic Press.

Giovacchini, P. L. (1969). The influence of interpretation upon schizophrenic patients. *International Journal of Psychoanalysis, 50*: 179–186.

Giovacchini, P. L. (1972). Interpretation and the definition of the analytic setting. In: P. L. Giovacchini (Ed.), *Tactics and Techniques in Psychoanalytic Therapy, Vol. 2* (pp. 5–94). New York: Jason Aronson.

Glover, E. (1931). The therapeutic effect of inexact interpretation. *International Journal of Psychoanalysis, 12*: 397–418.

Glover, E. (1955). *The Technique of Psychoanalysis*. New York: International Universities Press.

Green, A. (2000). The intrapsychic and the intrasubjective in psychoanalysis. *Psychoanalytic Quarterly, 69*: 1–39.

Green, N., & Solnit, A. J. (1964). Reactions to the threatened loss of a child: A vulnerable child syndrome. *Pediatrics, 34*: 58–66.

Greenson, R. R. (1958). Variations in classical psychoanalytic technique. *International Journal of Psychoanalysis, 39*: 200–201.

Greenson, R. R. (1967). *The Technique and Practice of Psychoanalysis.* New York: International Universities Press.

Greenspan, S. I. (1997). *The Growth of the Mind and the Endangered Origins of Intelligence.* Cambridge, MA: Perseus.

Gülüm, İ. V., & Soygüt, G. (2021). Limited reparenting as a corrective emotional experience in schema therapy: A preliminary task analysis. *Psychotherapy Research, 32*: 1–14.

Hamilton, J. W. (1969). Object loss, dreaming and creativity: The poetry of John Keats. *Psychoanalytic Study of the Child, 24*: 488–531.

Hamilton, J. W. (1979). Joseph Conrad: His development as an artist, 1889–1910. *Psychoanalytic Study of the Child, 8*: 277–329.

Harley, M., & Weil, A. (1979). Introduction. In: *Selected Papers of Margaret S. Mahler, Volume 1: Infantile Psychosis and Early Contributions* (pp. ix–xx). New York: Jason Aronson.

Hartzband, P., & Groopman, J. (2011). The new language of medicine. *New England Journal of Medicine, 365*: 1372–1373.

Hartzband, P., & Groopman, J. (2016). Medical taylorism. *New England Journal of Medicine, 374*: 106–108.

Hauke, W., Schwarzkopf, W., & Berberich, G. (2019). Annäherung von verhaltenstherapeutischen und psychodynamischen Konzepten am Beispiel der Zwangsstörung. *Psychodynamische Psychotherapie: Forum Der Tiefenpsychologisch Fundierten Psychotherapie, 18*: 43–54.

Heath, S. (1991). *Dealing with the Therapist's Vulnerability to Depression.* Northvale, NJ: Jason Aronson.

Hendrickson, B. (2015). Neo-shamans, curanderismo and scholars: Metaphysical blending in contemporary Mexican American folk healing. *Nova Religio: Journal of Alternative and Emergent Religions, 19*: 25–44.

Hoffer, A. (1985). Towards a definition of neutrality. *Journal of the American Psychoanalytic Association, 31*: 771–795.

Hollander, N. C. (2009). When not knowing allies with destructiveness: Global warning and psychoanalytic ethical non-neutrality. *International Journal of Applied Psychoanalytic Studies, 6*: 1–11.

Horney, K. (1967). *Feminine Psychology.* New York: W. W. Norton.

Inderbitzin, L. B., & Levy, S. T. (1990). Unconscious fantasy: A reconsideration of the concept. *Journal of the American Psychoanalytic Association, 38*: 113–130.

Jacobson, E. (1954). Transference problems in the psychoanalytic treatment of severely depressive patients. *Journal of the American Psychoanalytic Association, 2*: 595–606.

Jacobson, E. (1964). *The Self and the Object World*. New York: International Universities Press.

Janov, A. (1970). *The Primal Scream: Primal Therapy: The Cure for Neurosis*. New York: G. P. Putnam's Sons.

Johnson, R., Persad, G., & Sisti, D. (2014). The Tarasoff rule: The implications of interstate variation and gaps in professional training. *Journal of the American Academy of Psychiatry and the Law, 42*: 469–477.

Kaluzeviciute, G. (2020). Social media and its impact on therapeutic relationships. *British Journal of Psychotherapy, 36*: 303–320. https://doi.org/10.1111/bjp.12545

Kanner, L. (1942). *Child Psychiatry*. Springfield, IL: Thomas.

Katz, D. A., Kaplan, M., & Stromberg, S. E. (2012). A national survey of candidates: I. Demographics, practice patterns, and satisfaction with training. *Journal of the American Psychoanalytic Association, 60*(1): 71–96.

Kernberg, O. F. (1975). *Borderline Conditions and Pathological Narcissism*. New York. Jason Aronson.

Kernberg, O. F. (1976). Technical considerations in the treatment of borderline personality organization. *Journal of the American Psychoanalytic Association, 30*: 795–829.

Kernberg, O. F. (1980). *Internal World and External Reality: Object Relations Theory Applied* (Revised). New York: Jason Aronson.

Kernberg, O. F. (1984a). *Severe Personality Disorders: Psychotherapeutic Strategies*. New Haven, CT: Yale University Press.

Kernberg, O. F. (1984b). The couch at sea: Psychoanalytic studies of group and organizational leadership. *International Journal of Group Psychotherapy, 34*: 5–23.

Kernberg, O. F. (1988). Object relations theory in clinical practice. *Psychoanalytic Quarterly, 57*: 481–504.

Kernberg, O. F. (1998). *Ideology, Conflict, and Leadership in Groups and Organizations*. New Haven, CT: Yale University Press.

Kernberg, O. F. (2001). Recent developments in the technical approaches of English-language psychoanalytic schools. *Psychoanalytic Quarterly, 70*: 519–547.

Kernberg, O. F. (2003a). Sanctioned political violence: A psychoanalytic view—Part 1. *International Journal of Psychoanalysis, 84*: 683–698.

Kernberg, O. F. (2003b). Sanctioned political violence: A psychoanalytic view—Part 2. *International Journal of Psychoanalysis, 84*: 953–968.

Kestenberg, J. S. (1982). A psychological assessment based on analysis of a survivor's child. In: M. S. Bergmann & M. E. Jucovy (Eds.), *Generations of the Holocaust* (pp. 158–177). New York: Columbia University Press.

Kestenberg, J. S., & Brenner, I. (1996). *The Last Witness*. Washington, DC: American Psychiatric Press.

Kittay, E. F. (1984). Rereading Freud on "femininity" or why not womb envy? *Women's Studies International Forum, 7*: 385–391.

Klautau, P., & Coelho, N. (2013). On psychic reality and neutrality: Empathy and the work of construction in countertransference. *International Forum of Psychoanalysis, 22*: 142–148.

Klein, M. (1932). *Psycho-Analysis of Children*. London: International Psychoanalytic Library.

Klein, M. (1946). Notes on some schizoid mechanisms. *International Journal of Psychoanalysis, 27*: 99–110.

Kogan, I. (1995). *The Cry of Mute Children: A Psychoanalytic Perspective of the Second Generation of the Holocaust*. London: Free Association.

Kohut, H. (1971). *The Analysis of the Self: A Systematic Approach to the Psychoanalytic Treatment of Narcissistic Personality Disorders*. New York: International Universities Press.

König, K., Lindner, W.-V., & Foulkes, P. (1994). *Psychoanalytic Group Therapy*. Northvale, NJ: Jason Aronson.

Kramer, S., & Rudolph, J. (1980). The latency stage. In: S. I. Greenspan & G. H. Pollack (Eds.), *The Course of Life, Volume II: Latency, Adolescence, and Youth* (pp. 109–119). Adelphi, MD: National Institute of Mental Health.

Kris, A. (1982). *Free Associations*. New Haven, CT: Yale University Press.

Kutter, P. (1982). *Basic Aspects of Psychoanalytic Group Therapy*. London: Routledge.

Laplanche, J., & Pontalis, J.-B. (1973). *The Language of Psycho-Analysis*. D. Nicholson-Smith (Trans.). New York: W. W. Norton.

Laub, D., & Auerhahn, N. C. (1993). Knowing and not knowing massive psychic trauma: Forms of traumatic memory. *International Journal of Psychoanalysis, 74*: 287–302.

Legg, C., & Sherick, I. (1976). The replacement child—A developmental tragedy: Some preliminary comments. *Child Psychiatry and Human Development, 7*: 79–97.

Lehtonen, J. (2003).The dream between neuroscience and psychoanalysis: Has feeding an infant an impact on brain function and the capacity to create dream images in infants? *Psychoanalysis in Europe, 57*: 175–182.

Leonidaki, V. (2021). Moving beyond a single-model philosophy: Integrating relational therapies in front-line psychological therapy services in England. *Journal of Psychotherapy Integration, 31*: 70–85.

Levy, S. T. (1984). *Principles of Interpretation*. New York: Jason Aronson.

Lin, C.-H., Hsieh, Y.-J., & Sun, C.-T. (2008). Practice survey of counseling psychologists in Taiwan. *Chinese Journal of Guidance and Counseling, 23*: 117–145.

Lin, L., Nigrinis, A., Christidis, P., & Stamm, K. (2015). *Demographics of the U.S. Psychology Workforce: Findings from the American Community Survey (Center for Workforce Studies)*. Washington, DC: American Psychological Association.

Lipson, G. S., & Mills, M. J. (1998). Stalking, erotomania, and the Tarasoff cases. In: J. R. Meloy (Ed.), *The Psychology of Stalking: Clinical and Forensic Perspectives* (pp. 257–273). Cambridge, MA: Academic Press.

Lloyd, C., King, R., Bassett, H., Sandland, S., & Savige, G. (2001). Patient, client or consumer? A survey of preferred terms. *Australasian Psychiatry, 9*: 321–324.

Loewald, H. W. (1960). On the therapeutic action of psychoanalysis. *International Journal of Psychoanalysis, 41*: 16–33.

Leowald, H. W. (1988). On the mode of therapeutic action of psychoanalytic psychotherapy. In: *How Does Treatment Help? On the Modes of Therapeutic Action of Psychoanalytic Psychotherapy* (pp. 51–59). Madison, CT: International Universities Press.

Loewenstein, R. M. (1951). The problem of interpretation. *Psychoanalytic Quarterly, 20*: 1–14.

Loewenstein, R. M. (1958). Remarks on some variations in psychoanalytic technique. *International Journal of Psychoanalysis, 39*: 202–210.

Lombardi, R. (2020). Corona virus, social distancing, and the body in psychoanalysis. *Journal of the American Psychoanalytic Association, 68*: 455–462.

Ludwig-Körner, C. (2021). Psychoanalytikerin als Beruf—eine wechselvolle Geschichte (Psychoanalyst as profession for women—An eventful history). *Forum der Psychoanalyse: Zeitschrift für klinische Theorie & Praxis, 37*: 165–181.

Mahler, M. S. (1958). On two crucial phases of integration of the sense of identity: Separation–individuation and bisexual identity. *Journal of the American Psychoanalytic Association, 6*: 136–139.

Mahler, M. S. (1968). *On Human Symbiosis and the Vicissitudes of Individuation*. New York: International Universities Press.

McWilliams, N. (1999). *Psychoanalytic Case Formulation*. New York: Guilford.

Mead, M. (1949). *Male and Female: A Study of the Sexes in a Changing World*. New York: William Morrow.

Menninger, K. A. (1958). *Theory of Psychoanalytic Technique*. New York: Harper & Row.

Mills, J. (2015). Psychotherapist–patient privilege, record keeping, and maintaining psychotherapy case notes in professional practice: The need for ethical and policy reform. *Canadian Journal of Counselling and Psychotherapy, 49*: 96–113.

Mitchell, J. (1974). *Psychoanalysis and Feminism*. New York: Vintage.

Mitchell, S. A. (1988). *Relational Concepts in Psychoanalysis: An Integration*. Cambridge, MA: Harvard University Press.

Mitchell, S. A. (2000). *Relationality: From Attachment to Intersubjectivity*. Hillsdale, NJ: Analytic Press.

Moore, B. E., & Fine, B. D. (Eds.) (1990). *Psychoanalytic Terms and Concepts*. New Haven, CT: Yale University Press.

Moran, M. (2022). Study shows declining trend in psychotherapy by psychiatrists. *Psychiatric News, 57*: 34–35.

Musk, E. (2022, May 31). Remote work is no longer acceptable [Tweet]. Twitter. https://twitter.com/TechEmails/status/1531994582669348864/photo/1

Nakamura, K., Iwakabe, S., & Heim, N. (2022). Connecting in-session corrective emotional experiences with postsession therapeutic changes: A systematic case study. *Psychotherapy, 59*: 63–73.

Naseem, A., Balon, R., & Khan, S. (2001). Customer, client, consumer, recipient, or patient. *Annals of Clinical Psychiatry, 13*: 239–240.

Novick, J., & Kelly, K. (1970). Projection and externalization. *Psychoanalytic Study of the Child, 25*: 69–95.

Ogas, O., & Gaddam, S. (2011). *A Billion Wicked Thoughts: What the World's Largest Experiment Reveals about Human Desire*. New York: Dutton/Penguin.

Olinick, S. (1980). *The Psychotherapeutic Instrument*. New York: Jason Aronson.

Olos, L., & Hoff, E.-H. (2006). Gender ratios in European psychology. *European Psychologist, 11*: 1–11.

Parens, H. (2007). *Development of Aggression in Early Childhood*. Lanham, MD: Rowman & Littlefield.

Peck, S. (2021). Corrective emotional experiences: History, functions, and applications (2021-65614-111; Issues 12-B). Ann Arbor, MI: ProQuest Information & Learning.

Perls, F., Hefferline, R. F., & Goodman, P. (1965). *Gestalt Therapy*. New York: Dell.

Pine, F. (1997). *Diversity and Direction in Psychoanalytic Technique*. New Haven, CT: Yale University Press.

Pines, M., & Schermer, V. (1994). *Primitive Affects and Object Relations in Group Psychotherapy*. London: Routledge.

Plank, E. M., & Plank, R. (1978). Children and death: As seen through art and autobiographies. *Psychoanalytic Study of the Child*, 33(1): 593–620.

Poland, W. S. (1984). On the analyst's neutrality. *Journal of the American Psychoanalytic Association*, 32: 283–299.

Pollock, G. H. (1975). On mourning, immortality, and utopia. *Journal of the American Psychoanalytic Association*, 23(2): 334–362.

Poznanski, E. O. (1972). The "replacement child": A saga of unresolved parental grief. *Behavioral Pediatrics*, 81: 1190–1193.

Prince, R. N. (2021). Pandemic psychoanalysis. *American Journal of Psychoanalysis*, 81: 467–479.

Purhonen, M., Kilpeläinen-Lees, R., Valkonen-Korhonen, M., Karhu, J., & Lehtonen, J. (2005). Four-month-old infants process own mother's voice faster than unfamiliar voices: Electrical signs of sensitization in infant brain. *Cognitive Brain Research*, 3: 627–633.

Rangell, L. (2000). Psychoanalysis at the millennium: A unitary theory. *Psychoanalytic Psychology*, 17: 451–466.

Rim, J. I., Cabaniss, D. L., & Topor, D. (2020). Psychotherapy tracks in US general psychiatry residency programs: A proxy for trends in psychotherapy education. *Academic Psychiatry*, 44: 423–426.

Ritchie, C. W., Hayes, D., & Ames, D. J. (2000). Patient or client? The opinions of people attending a psychiatric clinic. *Psychiatric Bulletin*, 24: 447–450.

Rogers, C. R. (1951). *Client-centered Therapy: Its Current Practice, Implications, and Theory*. Boston, MA: Houghton Mifflin.

Romero, G. A. (Director). (1968, October 4). *Night of the Living Dead* [Horror, Thriller]. Image Ten.

Rosenfeld, D. (1992). *The Psychotic: Aspects of the Personality*. London: Karnac.

Rosenfeld, H. A. (1965). *Psychotic States: A Psychoanalytic Approach*. London: Hogarth.

Rudenstine, S., Wright, L., Morales, A.-M., & Tuber, S. (2018). The value of integration: Psychoanalytic psychotherapy meets ego psychology in a psychotherapy group for children. *Journal of Infant, Child & Adolescent Psychotherapy*, 17: 346–363.

Rutan, J. S., Stone, W. N., & Shay, J. J. (2014). *Psychodynamic Group Psychotherapy* (5th ed.). New York: Guilford.

Rycroft, C. (1972). *A Clinical Dictionary of Psychoanalysis*. London: Penguin.

Schill, M. A. (2004). Analytic neutrality, anonymity, abstinence, and elective self-disclosure. *Journal of the American Psychoanalytic Association*, 52: 151–187.

Schlesinger, H. (2003). *The Texture of Treatment: On the Matter of Psychoanalytic Technique*. Hillsdale, NJ: Analytic Press.

Schultz-Venrath, U., Brand, T., Euler, S., & Fuhrländer, S. (2012). Mental-isierungsbasierte Therapie für Persönlichkeitsstörungen—Ein (neues) Paradigma für behavoriale und psychodynamische Psychotherapien? *Schweizer Archiv für Neurologie und Psychiatrie, 163*: 179–186.

Schützenberger, A. A. (1998). *The Ancestor Syndrome: Transgenerational Psychotherapy and the Hidden Links in the Family Tree.* New York: Routledge.

Segal, H. (1973). *Introduction to the Work of Melanie Klein.* New York: Basic Books.

Shakespeare, W. (1623). *As You Like It.* J. Dusinberre (Ed.). The Arden Shakespeare. London: Thomas Learning, 2006.

Shanok, A. F. (2015). Driving me sane: Integrating CBT and relational psychodynamic psychotherapy. In: J. Bresler & K. Starr (Eds.), *Relational Psychoanalysis and Psychotherapy Integration: An Evolving Synergy.* New York: Routledge/Taylor & Francis.

Shapiro, T. (1984). On neutrality. *Journal of the American Psychoanalytic Association, 32*: 269–282.

Sharpe, E. F. (1950). *Collected Papers on Psycho-analysis.* M. Brierley (Ed.). London: Hogarth.

Shoshani, M., & Shoshani, B. (2021). *Timeless Grandiosity and Eroticized Contempt: Technical Challenges Posed by Cases of Narcissism and Perversion.* Bicester, UK: Phoenix.

Simons, R. C. (2003). The lawsuit revisited. *Journal of the American Psychoanalytic Association, 51*(Suppl): 247–271.

Sluzki, C. E. (2000). Patients, clients, consumers: The politics of words. *Families, Systems, & Health, 18*: 347–352.

Spitz, R. (1965). *The First Year of Life: A Psychoanalytic Study of Normal and Deviant Development of Object Relations.* New York: International Universities Press.

Stern, D. N. (1985). *The Interpersonal World of the Infant: A View from Psychoanalysis and Developmental Psychology.* New York: Basic Books.

Stone, L. (1954). The widening scope of indications for psychoanalysis. *Journal of the American Psychoanalytic Association, 2*: 567–594.

Stone, L. (1961). *The Psychoanalytic Situation.* New York: International Universities Press.

Streltzer, J. (Ed.) (2017). *Culture and Psychopathology: A Guide to Clinical Assessment.* New York: Routledge/Taylor & Francis.

Sullivan, H. S. (1962). *Schizophrenia as a Human Process.* New York: W. W. Norton.

Tadmon, D., & Olfson, M. (2022). Trends in outpatient psychotherapy provision by US psychiatrists: 1996–2016. *American Journal of Psychiatry*, *179*: 110–121.

Tähkä, V. (1993). *Mind and Its Treatment: A Psychoanalytic Approach*. Madison, CT: International Universities Press.

Torrey, E. F. (2011). Patients, clients, consumers, survivors et al.: What's in a name? *Schizophrenia Bulletin*, *37*: 456–468.

Valenstein, A. (1973). On attachment to painful feelings and the negative therapeutic reaction. *Psychoanalytic Study of the Child*, *28*: 365–392.

Veloce, L. F., Murkar, A., Klauck, M., DeCicco, T., & Nesbitt, D. (2019). The effects of emotional salience on the day-residue and dream-lag effects. *International Journal of Dream Research*, *12*: 62–69.

Volkan, K. (1994a). Psychopathology, groups, and group leaders: A psychoanalytic perspective. *Vision/Action*, *13*: 19–24.

Volkan, K. (1994b). *Dancing Among the Maenads: The Psychology of Compulsive Drug Use*. Bern, Switzerland: Peter Lang.

Volkan, K. (2013a). Some considerations on zombies. *Journal of Social Sciences Research*, *1*: 58–69.

Volkan, K. (2013b). A psychoanalytic view of the Sangha: Group functioning in Mahayana and Tibetan Buddhism. *Asian Journal of Humanities and Social Studies*, *1*: 47–54.

Volkan, K. (2014). Whale wars: A somewhat psychoanalytic review. *Asian Journal of Humanities and Social Studies*, *2*: 616–620.

Volkan, K. (2016). Personality disorders: A review of the current state of knowledge. *Webmedcentral Psychology*, *7*: 1–16.

Volkan, K. (2020a). Delusional misidentification syndromes: Psychopathology and culture. *Journal of Health and Medical Sciences*, *3*: 288–301.

Volkan, K. (2020b). Encounter with the demonic: Western, Eastern, and object relations approaches. *Psychology*, *11*: 1454–1470.

Volkan, K. (2021a). Bunkers, bubbles, monuments, and walls: Pathological narcissism, Nazi Germany, and Donald Trump. *European Journal of Psychoanalysis*, *14*: 1–21.

Volkan, K. (2021b). Hoarding and animal hoarding: Psychodynamic and transitional aspects. *Psychodynamic Psychiatry*, *49*: 24–47.

Volkan, K., & Volkan, V. D. (2022). *Schizophrenia: Science, Psychoanalysis, and Culture*. Bicester, UK: Phoenix.

Volkan, V. D. (1976). *Primitive Internalized Object Relations: A Clinical Study of Schizophrenic, Borderline and Narcissistic Patients*. New York: International Universities Press.

Volkan, V. D. (1979). *Cyprus—War and Adaptation: A Psychoanalytic History of Two Ethnic Groups in Conflict.* Charlottesville, VA: University Press of Virginia.

Volkan, V. D. (1981). *Linking Objects and Linking Phenomena: A Study of the Forms, Symptoms, Metapsychology and Therapy of Complicated Mourning.* New York: International Universities Press.

Volkan, V. D. (1987). *Six Steps in the Treatment of Borderline Personality Organization.* Northvale, NJ: Jason Aronson.

Volkan, V. D. (1988). *The Need to Have Enemies and Allies: From Clinical Practice to International Relationships.* Northvale, NJ: Jason Aronson.

Volkan, V. D. (1995). *The Infantile Psychotic Self: Understanding and Treating Schizophrenics and Other Difficult Patients.* Northvale, NJ: Jason Aronson.

Volkan, V. D. (1997). *Bloodlines: From Ethnic Pride to Ethnic Terrorism.* New York: Farrar, Straus & Giroux.

Volkan, V. D. (2004). Actualized unconscious fantasies and "therapeutic play" in adults' analyses: Further study of these concepts. In: A. Laine (Ed.), *Power of Understanding: Essays in Honour of Veikko Tähkä* (pp. 119–141). London: Karnac.

Volkan, V. D. (2005). *Fanustaki İnsanlar (People in the Bubble).* Istanbul, Turkey: Alfa.

Volkan, V. D. (2006a). Grossgruppen und ihre politischen Fürermitnarzisstischer Personlichkeitsorganisation. In: O. F. Kernberg & H.-P. Hartmann (Eds.), *Grunlagen-Störungsbilder – Therapie* (pp. 205–227). Stuttgart, Germany: Schattauer.

Volkan, V. D. (2006b). *Killing in the Name of Identity: A Study of Bloody Conflicts.* Durham, NC: Pitchstone.

Volkan, V. D. (2010). *Psychoanalytic Technique Expanded: A Textbook on Psychoanalytic Treatment.* Istanbul, Turkey: Oa.

Volkan, V. D. (2013). *Enemies on the Couch: A Psychopolitical Journey Through War and Peace.* Durham, NC: Pitchstone.

Volkan, V. D. (2014). *Animal Killer: Transmission of War Trauma from One Generation to the Next.* London: Karnac.

Volkan, V. D. (2018). *Blind Trust: Large Groups and Their Leaders in Times of Crisis and Terror.* Durham, NC: Pitchstone.

Volkan, V. D. (2019a). *Ghosts in the Human Psyche: The Story of a "Muslim Armenian."* Bicester, UK: Phoenix.

Volkan, V. D. (2019b). *A Nazi Legacy: Depositing, Transgenerational Transmission, Dissociation, and Remembering Through Action.* London: Karnac.

Volkan, V. D. (2020). *Large-Group Psychology: Racism, Who Are We Now? Societal Divisions and Narcissistic Leaders.* Bicester, UK: Phoenix.

Volkan, V. D. (2021a). *Therapeutic Approaches to Varied Psychoanalytic Cases.* Cheng Hao (Trans.).Taiwan: PsyGarden.

Volkan, V. D. (2021b). *Sexual Addiction: Psychoanalytic Concepts and the Art of Supervision.* Bicester, UK: Phoenix.

Volkan, V. D. (2021c). Sixteen analysands' and large groups' reactions to the COVID-19 pandemic. *International Journal of Applied Psychoanalytic Studies, 18*: 159–168.

Volkan, V. D., & Ast, G. (1992). *Eine Borderline-Therapie: Strukturelle und Objektbeziehungskonflikte in der Psychoanalyse der Borderline-Persönlichkeitsorganisation.* Göttingen, Germany: Vandenhoeck & Ruprecht.

Volkan, V. D., & Ast, G. (1994). *Spektrum des Narzißmus:Eine klinische Studie des gesunden Narzißmus, des narzißtisch-masochistischen Charakters, der narzißtischen Persönlichkeitsorganisaticn, des malignen Narzißmus und des erfolgreichen Narzißmus.* Göttingen, Germany: Vandenhoeck & Ruprecht.

Volkan, V. D., & Ast, G. (1997). *Siblings in the Unconscious and Psychopathology.* Madison, CT: International Universities Press.

Volkan, V. D., & Ast, G. (2001). Curing Gitta's "leaking body": Actualized unconscious fantasies and therapeutic play. *Journal of Clinical Psychoanalysis, 10*: 567–606.

Volkan, V. D., Ast, G., & Greer, W. F. (2002). *The Third Reich in the Unconscious: Transgenerational Transmission and Its Consequences.* New York: Brunner-Routledge.

Volkan, V. D., & Fowler, C. (2009). *Searching for the Perfect Woman: The Story of a Complete Psychoanalysis.* Northvale, NJ: Jason Aronson.

Volkan, V. D., & Itzkowitz, N. (1984). *The Immortal Atatürk: A Psychobiography.* Chicago, IL: University of Chicago Press.

Volkan, V. D., & Javakhishvili, J. D. (2022). Invasion of Ukraine: Observations on leader–followers relationships. *American Journal of Psychoanalysis, 82*: 189–209.

Waelder, R. (1936). The principle of multiple function: Observations on multiple determination. *Psychoanalytic Quarterly, 5*: 45–62.

Waheed, N. (2013). *Salt.* Scotts Valley, CA: CreateSpace Independent Publishing Platform.

Wakefield, J. C., & Baer, J. C. (2010). The cognitivization of psychoanalysis: Toward an integration of psychodynamic and cognitive theories. In: W. Borden (Ed.), *Reshaping Theory in Contemporary Social Work: Toward a Critical Pluralism in Clinical Practice* (pp. 51–80). New York: Columbia University Press.

Wallerstein, R. S. (1988). One psychoanalysis or many? *International Journal of Psychoanalysis, 69*: 5–21.

Wallwork, E. (2005). Ethics in psychoanalysis. In: E. S. Person, A. M. Cooper, & G. O. Gabbard (Eds.), *The Textbook of Psychoanalysis* (pp. 281–297). Washington, DC: American Psychiatric Publishing.

Weigert, E. (1954). The importance of flexibility in psychoanalytic technique. *Journal of the American Psychoanalytic Association, 2*: 702–710.

Weisbord, M. R. (1987). *Productive Workplaces*. New York: Jossey-Bass.

Werman, D. S. (1984).The premature transference. Paper presented at the American Psychoanalytic Association Meeting, San Diego, California, May 16–20.

Werner, H., & Kaplan, B. (1963). *Symbol Formation*. New York: Wiley.

Winnicott, D. W. (1965). *The Maturational Processes and the Facilitating Environment*. New York: International Universities Press.

Winnicott, D. W. (1992). *Through Pediatrics to Psycho-Analysis: Collected Papers*. New York: Brunner/Mazel.

Wolfenstein, M. (1966). How mourning is possible. *Psychoanalytic Study of the Child, 21*: 93–123.

Wolfenstein, M. (1969). Loss, rage and repetition. *Psychoanalytic Study of the Child, 24*: 432–460.

Wolfenstein, M. (1973). The image of the lost parent. *Psychoanalytic Study of the Child, 28*: 433–456.

Yalom, I. D. (2009). *Staring at the Sun: Overcoming the Terror of Death*. New York: Jossey-Bass.

Zepf, S. (2015). Penisneid und weiblicher Ödipuskomplex: Ein Plädoyer für die Wiederaufnahme einerwirkungsvollen Debatte. *Zeitschrift für psychoanalytische Theorie und Praxis, 30*: 65–92.

Zetzel, E. (1956). Current concepts of transference. *International Journal of Psychoanalysis, 37*: 369–375.

Index